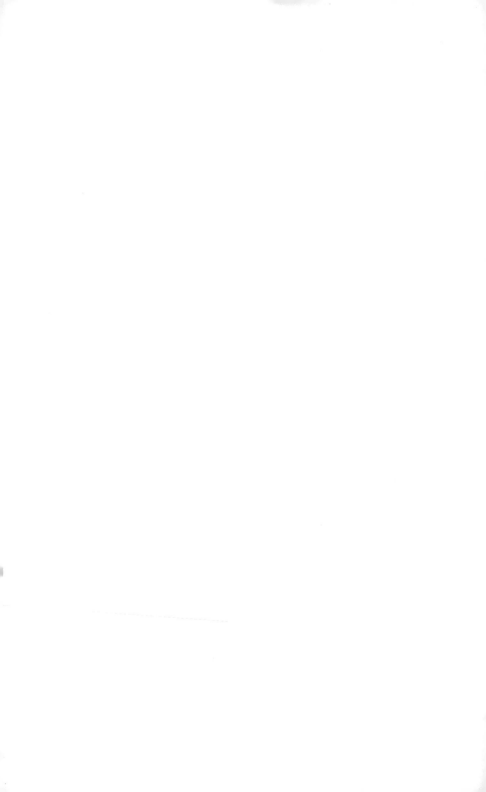

Panoramic Radiology

Quintessentials of Dental Practice – 20
Imaging – 2

Panoramic Radiology

By
Vivian E Rushton
John Rout

Editor-in-Chief: Nairn H F Wilson
Editor Imaging: Keith Horner

Quintessence Publishing Co. Ltd.
London, Berlin, Chicago, Paris, Milan, Barcelona, Istanbul,
São Paulo, Tokyo, New Delhi, Moscow, Prague, Warsaw

British Library Cataloguing-in Publication Data

Rushton, V. E.
  Panoramic radiology. - (Quintessentials of dental practice: 20.
  Imaging; 2)
  1. Teeth - Radiography 2. Radiography, Panoramic
  I. Title II. Rout, John
  617.6´07572

ISBN 1850970807

Copyright © 2006 Quintessence Publishing Co. Ltd., London

ISBN 1-85097-080-7

Foreword

Panoramic radiology is extensively used in everyday clinical practice. It is therefore important that both existing and future practitioners are fully familiar with this imaging technique, the interpretation of panoramic images and very importantly, the indications and clinical justifications for such extraoral imaging. Practitioners using panoramic radiology must also have knowledge of relevant radiation doses, risks to patients and quality assurance protocols.

Panoramic Radiology, Volume 20 in the timely *Quintessentials for General Dental Practitioners* series, addresses all of these issues and, in addition, gives a great deal of practical guidance on panoramic radiology as it ought to be applied by practitioners. As with all forms of radiological examination each and every panoramic image should have a net benefit for the patient, with the exposure to ionising radiation having been optimised for the intended purpose. This excellent, succinct, generously illustrated book will assist practitioners in satisfying this requirement in relation to panoramic radiology.

As all members of the dental team should play their respective parts in ensuring the safe, appropriate and effective use of panoramic imaging, this book should find its way into the practice environment for all to study and use to good effect. An excellent addition to all practitioner and practice collections of reference texts.

Nairn Wilson
Editor-in-Chief

Acknowledgements

We would like to thank our respective families and colleagues for their help and encouragement during the writing of this book and also those patients whose clinical radiographs are integral to a book of this nature.

Contents

Chapter 1
Panoramic Radiography: History and Future Development

Aim

The aim of the chapter is to present an overview of the development of dental panoramic radiography during the past century.

Outcome

After studying this chapter, the reader should have a clear understanding of the historical development of panoramic radiography and of the more recent technological advances in panoramic image production, including digital imaging techniques.

Introduction

Dental panoramic radiography is a radiographic technique that produces an image of both jaws and their respective dentitions on a single extraoral radiographic film. The development of panoramic radiographic equipment represented a major innovation in the field of dental imaging as, prior to this, dental radiographic images consisted solely of intraoral and oblique lateral projections of the jaws taken using a conventional dental x-ray set.

Today panoramic radiographic equipment is found routinely both within most hospital radiology departments and in a high proportion of general dental practices. It has been estimated that around 60% of United Kingdom dentists have direct access to panoramic equipment. A similar level of use has been reported in other parts of the industrialised world.

Development of the Technique

In the early part of the 20th century, many researchers were developing techniques using movement of the x-ray tube and the film in order to visualise structures or foreign bodies (particularly bullets) situated within the patient. Andre Bocage, a French researcher, was the originator of the principles of body-section imaging. In Bocage's seminal work, patented in 1922, the author mentions the possibility of imaging curved surfaces such as the jaws.

Further interest in this field of research did not resurface for another 20 years and resulted in the development of x-ray equipment using two quite different radiographic techniques to produce an overall image of the jaws. One group of researchers developed a small x-ray source which, when positioned intraorally, would directly expose an x-ray film moulded to the outside of the patient's face. The other group relied upon the production of a tomographic image of the jaws with the tube positioned extraorally, combined with either an intraorally or an extraorally positioned film.

Panoramic Equipment Using an Intraoral Source of Radiation

Bouchacourt first proposed the possibility of using an intraoral source of radiation to image the jaws as early as 1898. This concept was finally developed almost half a century later when two separate groups of researchers applied for patents to develop intraoral panoramic equipment. These were, in 1943, the German company of Koch and Sterzel (Fig 1-1), followed in 1951 by the Swiss researcher Dr. Walter Ott. Dr. Sydney Blackman, a British radi-

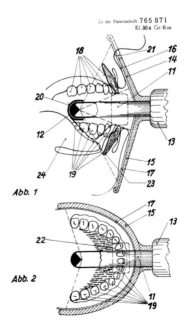

Fig 1-1 Patent issued to the Koch and Sterzel Aktiengesellschaft of Düsseldorf, Germany, for x-ray equipment capable of imaging body cavities. Horst Bergen is named as the inventor of the equipment.

ologist, modified the principles proposed by Dr. Ott, leading to the commercial development by Watson and Sons Ltd. of the 'Panograph' panoramic equipment (Fig 1-2).

Intraoral panoramic equipment used a cone-shaped anode located at the end of a thin rod (Fig 1-2) with a focal spot (the source of the x-ray beam) that was extremely small (ca. 0.1 mm) compared to conventional x-ray equipment. The intraoral technique had several inherent problems. It was extremely time-consuming, requiring separate exposures for both the maxilla and mandible (Fig 1-3). The technique also resulted in severe geometric distortion and, more importantly, delivered high doses of radiation to the oral tissues, notably the tongue. Paradoxically, these factors appeared not to have deterred the development of an intraoral panoramic unit that relied upon a radioactive isotope as its source of radiation. Fortunately, common sense prevailed and further experimentation with this type of intraoral panoramic equipment was rapidly curtailed, not least because of the obvious radiation risk but also the cost of the isotope.

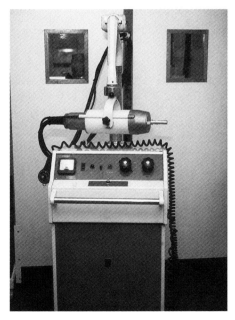

Fig 1-2 Panograph intraoral panoramic unit showing the slender x-ray tube.

3

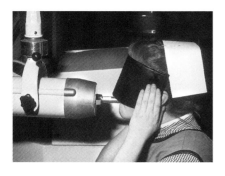

Fig 1-3 Panograph intraoral panoramic unit. Patient positioned with the anode intraorally and the maxillary film moulded to face.

Further development of the intraoral type of panoramic equipment centred upon improving patient comfort and reducing image distortion. An eccentric positioning of the x-ray tube was an attempt to improve the latter; however, the problems of geometric distortion proved insurmountable. Finally, the unacceptable dose level delivered by this type of equipment led to legislation within the United Kingdom recommending its withdrawal from clinical practice.

Panoramic Equipment Using an Extraoral Source of Radiation

The records of the American Patent Office show that in 1922, a patent was issued to A.F. Zulauf for 'Panoramic X-ray Apparatus' (Fig 1-4). The equipment used a rotational narrow beam x-ray technique that scanned either the upper or lower jaw with an intraorally positioned waterproofed lead–backed film packet to receive the image. The x-ray generator was moved manually around the patient on a mobile carriage supported on a U-shaped table using a preformed track. The researcher clearly understood the principles of image production but also its limitations. Zulauf stressed that the exact speed of movement was 'determined by experience and depends on the strength of the x-rays, the width of the collimator and its distance from the teeth being shadowgraphed'. While this patented design must qualify as the earliest example of rotational panoramic radiography, no further details concerning the subsequent development or the clinical use of the equipment have been found.

During the early 1930s, several researchers were active in pursuing and developing methods of imaging 'curved' structures such as the jaws. Numata proposed and discussed the principles of the panoramic technique as early as 1933, while at the same time constructing a suitable device for the clinical examination of the jaws. Numata's prototype used a very narrow collimated beam of x-ray photons, often referred to as a slit beam. The x-ray equipment

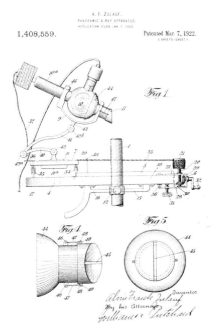

1,408,559.

A. F. ZULAUF.
PANORAMIC X-RAY APPARATUS.
APPLICATION FILED JAN. 7, 1920.

Patented Mar. 7, 1922.
2 SHEETS—SHEET 1

Fig 1-4 Patent of rotational x-ray equipment issued to A.F. Zulauf in 1922. Upper diagram is a side view elevation of the equipment. Figures 4 and 5 (on the patent document) are the top and front views, respectively, of the x-ray collimator.

rotated around the patient's head with the film positioned intraorally in the lingual sulcus.

Two researchers, Vieten and Heckmann, expounded the theoretical principles of imaging 'curved' structures without the superimposition of neighbouring structures. Both researchers experimented with a rotational slit beam technique to expose a film, but it was Olsson who refined the principles of an x-ray tube moving simultaneously to the detector, which is positioned behind the structure to be imaged.

In 1946, Dr. Yrjö Veli Paatero of the Institute of Dentistry, University of Helsinki, Finland, carried out similar work to that previously described by Olsson, although apparently unaware of this earlier research. The literature credits Paatero with developing and constructing the first working prototype of an extraoral rotational panoramic unit. The design of this unit was similar to that

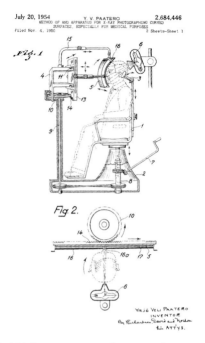

July 20, 1954   Y. V. PAATERO   2,684,446
METHOD OF AND APPARATUS FOR X-RAY PHOTOGRAPHING CURVED
SURFACES, ESPECIALLY FOR MEDICAL PURPOSES
Filed Nov. 4, 1950   2 Sheets—Sheet 1

Fig 1-5 Patent 2,684,446 for an apparatus for x-ray photographing curved surfaces, issued to YV Paatero in 1954. The schematic shows how the equipment relied upon a cog wheel (10) to move the cassette holder (14) along with the curved cassette (5). The stationary x-ray source (6) is easily seen as is the lead shield labelled 16. The crank (7) rotated the chair either by hand or via an electric motor.

proposed by Numata in 1933. Paatero's prototype positioned the film intra-orally, requiring a separate film for each jaw. The equipment used a stationary slit collimated x-ray beam which scanned the teeth and jaws by manually rotating the patients around the x-ray source as they sat in the dental chair.

Further research by Paatero in 1949 resulted in the development of a single axis or concentric rotational panoramic system. This system incorporated a curved extraoral film cassette (Fig 1-5) rather than the time-consuming and uncomfortable intraoral placement of the image receptor. The equipment continued to use a slit collimated x-ray beam with the patient and the curved extraoral film cassette rotating around a stationary x-ray source, with the film exposed through a vertical slit. The method of exposure consisted of rotation of the patient in front of a stationary x-ray tube as the film was translated behind the vertical slit to achieve a sequential exposure.

Meanwhile, in the early 1950s, two US researchers, Dr RJ Nelson and JW Kumpula, had begun to develop an experimental panoramic unit. Their equipment showed some similarities to that already developed by Paatero in that the film was positioned intraorally, but the tube and film movement was more complex. Collaboration between Paatero, Nelson and Kumpula began in 1950 at the University of Washington, resulting in the development of an automatic panoramic unit.

Paatero's single axis panoramic equipment often showed poor definition as well as a problematical overlap of teeth. Paatero overcame these problems by varying the position of the mandible relative to the single axis of rotation. Unfortunately, this modification lengthened the imaging procedure, as two separate exposures of each side of the jaw were needed. Nelson and Kumpula chose an alternative technique to resolve the problem, developing a double eccentric method in which the x-ray tube and film cassette revolved around the stationary patient.

In the USA, the impetus to further develop the panoramic technique was the perceived need of an imaging system that could rapidly record the dental status of large numbers of people, such as armed forces recruits and conscripts. Hudson and Kumpula were assigned to this task and began work to design a panoramic machine capable of meeting these prerequisites. The equipment developed, based upon the principle of double eccentric axes, proved extremely successful and the design was patented (Fig 1-6). This equipment later became commercially available, marketed as the 'Panorex'.

Paatero returned to Finland to concentrate on refining his own research (Figs 1-7, 1-8 and 1-9). He worked in collaboration with Dr. Sidney Blackman and Watson and Sons Ltd. to develop a commercial model of the pantomograph, known as the 'Rotograph' (Figs 1-10 and 1-11). By 1954, Paatero had published the theoretical basis for a new type of panoramic equipment that consisted of three rotational axes. The resultant image eliminated, to a large degree, the troublesome overlapping of the posterior teeth. The image became more of an orthoradial projection, i.e., one at right angles to the dental arch. This prompted Paatero to refer to his refined technique as orthoradial jaw pantomography, often shortened to 'orthopantomography'. Paatero carried out most of the preliminary experimentation on the orthopantomography in collaboration with Timo Nieminen, an outstanding engineer.

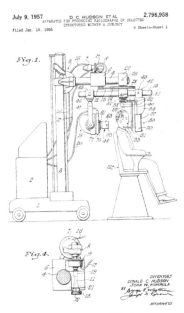

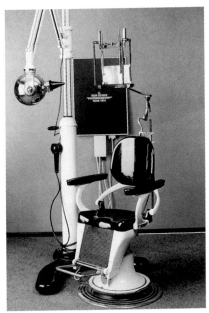

Fig 1-6 Patent 2,798,958 for panoramic equipment that was issued to Donald C Hudson and John W. Kumpula in 1956. This equipment was later commercially developed as the Panorex x-ray unit.

Fig 1-7 Paatero's prototype panoramic equipment dated 1951 (Kindly supplied by Instrumentarium Imaging, Tuusula, Finland.)

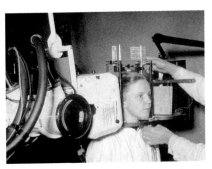

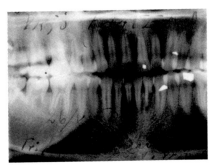

Fig 1-8 Dr. Paatero making fine adjustments to patient positioning. The device was subsequently installed in Helsinki University in 1951 (Kindly supplied by Instrumentarium Imaging, Tuusula, Finland.)

Fig 1-9 A reprint of the original panoramic film taken by Dr. Paatero on the 26th of December 1950.

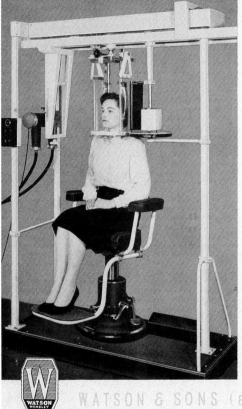

PUBLICATION № 580

WATSON

ROTAGRAPH

for Rotary Tomography of the Skull

WITH the aid of this apparatus, a radiograph of both the upper and lower jaws from one temporo-mandibular joint to the other, can be made in a single exposure on one film without causing the patient the slightest discomfort. The body of the mandible is " unfolded " and is shown in one plane, including both ascending rami. The examination may also be limited to the teeth-bearing area to demonstrate, for instance, unerupted teeth in the adolescent, and it has other valuable applications which will be referred to later.

The technique is the outcome of research by various workers including Dr. K. Heckmann[1], W. Watson[2], Dr. Yrjo V. Paatero[3] (whose term for the tomography of curved sections is " Pantomography ") and upon more recent work by Dr. Sydney Blackman[4] of the Royal Dental Hospital, under the auspices of St. George's Hospital, London.

The rotary tomograph is made by rotating the patient and a curved film simultaneously on their own axes and in opposite directions whilst a narrow beam of x-rays from a stationary x-ray tube passes through the area under examination. All points at equal distance have the same linear speed and thus remain stationary with respect to each other and thus receive the maximum exposure. Structures in front of and behind the selected plane have a different linear velocity and are thus not sharply projected on the film. They appear only as faint blurred marks.

Continued

A full mouth radiograph is made in 30 seconds without discomfort to the patient. The apparatus is also suitable for many other aspects of orthodontic radiography.

WATSON & SONS (ELECTRO-MEDICAL) LTD

Fig 1-10 A brochure advertising the Rotograph panoramic equipment.

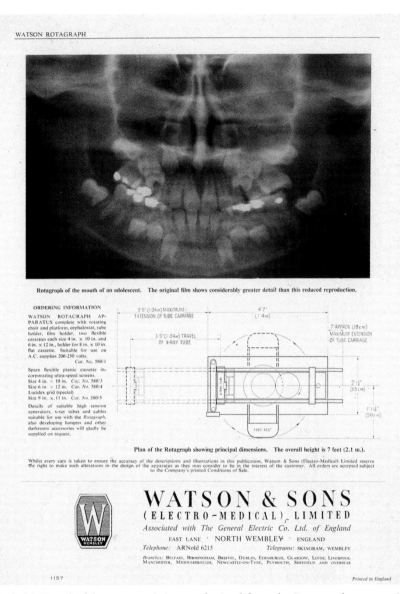

Fig 1-11 Detail of the panoramic image obtained from the Rotograph panoramic equipment. There was a much wider coverage of the jaws associated with early panoramic equipment.

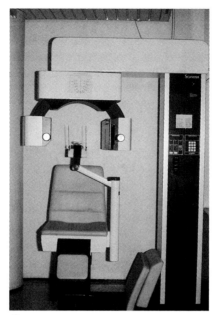

Fig 1-12 The Scanora® multi-functional tomographic unit (Kindly supplied by Mr. Martin Payne.)

Further Developments

Improvements in image production have centred upon refining rotational movement and determining the 'correct' form of the image layer. The development of a continuously moving rotational centre that follows an elliptical path has proved extremely successful. The type of rotational movement achieved by panoramic equipment has been found to be dependent upon the perceived shape and form of the dental arches. The necessity to describe mathematically the average curve of the dentition culminated in work by Nummikoski who determined arch shape to the fourth degree polynomial. Nummikoski's data have subsequently been incorporated into software controlling movement within several modern panoramic units.

Other technical refinements have been the introduction of constant potential generators, field limitation and the use of positioning lights to ensure correct positioning of the patient. Newer equipment offers the option of combining panoramic radiography with cross-sectional linear tomography programmes to allow an assessment of implant sites. A sophisticated machine of this type is the Scanora® (Fig 1-12), which employs the principles of narrow beam tomography and spiral tomography to produce high resolution cross-sectional images (Figs 1-13, 1-14 and 1-15). While these developments have made major contributions to panoramic radiology, it is the introduction of digital imaging that has made the most striking impact upon dentists.

Digital Imaging

The first x-ray images were recorded photographically, initially on glass plates and shortly afterwards using film, a system which has been refined and continues in use today, the process being referred to as radiography. An image captured this way is displayed as an analogue image (the radiograph).

A digital image, on the other hand, is made up of a series of numbers or digits created electronically and stored in a computer file. The image is fed to a computer, reconstructed as a series of shades of grey and displayed on a television monitor. This picture consists of a mosaic of numbers or digits arranged in a grid matrix, with each piece of the mosaic within the grid referred to as a pixel or picture element, as illustrated in Fig 1-16.

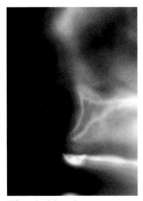 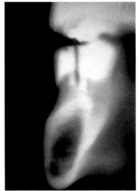 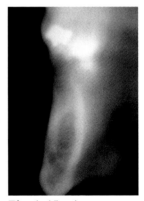

Fig 1-13 A transverse Scanora® cross-sectional image of the anterior maxilla showing alveolar bone and the nasal cavity (Kindly supplied by Mr. Martin Payne.)

Fig 1-14 A transverse Scanora® cross-sectional image of the mandible showing the position of the inferior dental canal. The vertical radiopaque lines represent metal markers in the localization stent (Kindly supplied by Mr. Martin Payne.)

Fig 1-15 A transverse Scanora® cross-sectional image of the mandible showing the mental canal (Kindly supplied by Mr. Martin Payne.)

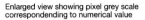

Enlarged view showing pixel grey scale corresponding to numerical value

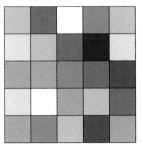

Numerical data of matrix grid following X-ray exposure

193	285	89	243	223
150	199	280	306	143
239	212	230	260	278
79	36	187	203	246
189	236	149	291	213

Fig 1-16 Diagramatic representation of pixels as numerical values and corresponding shades of grey.

Image resolution depends on the size of each pixel and the number in a given image: the more pixels, the clearer or sharper it appears. The grey scale also affects the image appearance. The eye can only discriminate up to about 30 shades of grey, but most modern desktop computers can store 256 (or more) shades of grey. This produces an image with smooth transitions between subtle or minor changes in grey shades.

There are two systems for obtaining a direct digital panoramic radiograph (DPR).

Charged Couple Device (CCD)
A charged couple device consists of a silicon chip which has an area divided into a grid. In order to obtain a digital image, x-ray photons are usually converted to light photons by means of a scintillator. The emitted light or, if a

13

scintillator is not used, the x-ray photons themselves interact with the CCD, storing electrons in the grid. The greater the number of photons striking a grid square, the larger the number of electrons that are stored. Each portion of the grid corresponds to a pixel. The grid is read, which produces levels of varying brightness depending on the number of stored electrons. The light emitted is converted into an electrical signal which is fed along a wire to the computer to be displayed on the screen.

More recently, a device similar to a CCD called a Complementary Metal Oxide Semiconductor Active Pixel Sensor (CMOS APS) has also been developed for medical imaging.

Photostimulable Phosphors (PSP)
The photostimulable phosphor (PSP) system consists of a reusable phosphor plate consists of europium-activated barium fluorohalide. When an x-ray photon interacts with the plate, it causes an electron to move out to a different orbit. It now has too much energy for that new orbit but is held in place until stimulated by a laser. As the electron moves back to its original orbit, it gives up its excess energy in the form of light (fluorescence), which is measured and displayed as an image.

Unlike the CCD system, there is no direct link from the sensor plate to the computer. The 'image' remains on the plate until it is transferred to the processing unit, which is connected to the computer. Here it is scanned by a laser beam to release the image for display on the television monitor. The image on the plate is cleared for reuse.

Whichever system is used, software packages are available to manipulate the digitised image by altering, for example, the contrast, brightness, grey scale inversion, noise reduction and subtraction. Images may be stored in computer files and a DPR will occupy several megabytes of disk space, unless image compression is used.

Conclusion
Panoramic radiography continues to evolve and use innovative technology for the benefit of the patient. It has developed from a theoretical possibility in 1898 to an established radiographic technique in the 21st century.

Acknowledgements

The authors would like to thank the following individuals for their help and advice during the writing of this chapter: Aimo Uimonen, Ouli Oksanen, Peter Hirschmann, Steven Webb and Henry Goodyear.

Further Reading

Grigg ERN. The trail of the invisible light; from X-Strahlen to Radio(bio)logy. Springfield Illinois: Charles C Thomas, 1965.

Langland OE, Langlais RP, McDavid WD and DelBalso AM. Panoramic Radiology. 2nd Edn. Philadelphia: Lea & Febiger, 1989.

Manson-Hing LR. Panoramic Dental Radiography. 1st Edn. Springfield Illinois: Charles C Thomas, 1976.

Webb S. From the watching of shadows. The origins of Radiological Tomography. Bristol: Adam Hilger, 1990.

Chapter 2
Dental Panoramic Radiographic Technique

Aim

The aims of this chapter are to outline the principles of panoramic image formation and the technique of dental panoramic radiography.

Outcome

After studying this chapter the reader should have an understanding of the basic concepts of dental panoramic image formation and the technique of obtaining a dental panoramic radiograph.

Introduction

Demonstrating the whole of both jaws on a single film is an advantage, particularly for assessing disorders too large to be recorded on intraoral radiographs or as a substitute for conditions requiring multiple intraoral films. If a Dental Panoramic Radiograph (DPR) is to be of optimal clinical value, it must be performed accurately and the resultant films correctly processed. The procedure of taking a DPR may seem reassuringly straightforward, but in fact it is technically exacting and requires attention to detail. Mastering the technique is made easier if you have a clear understanding of how the image is formed and of the image characteristics.

Panoramic Image Formation

The theory of panoramic image production is complex and beyond the remit of this book. However, a brief outline is provided, but for a more comprehensive account the reader is referred to other texts.

Obtaining a satisfactory single image of both jaws without distortion or superimposition of other structures is complicated because of their horseshoe shape. One solution to this problem is to record a curved slice that follows the shape of the jaws. The slice recorded in dental panoramic radiography is of variable width, being about 10 mm anteriorly and 25 mm posteriorly. The region imaged extends from the level of the orbital floor to the just below the lower border of the mandible. The curved object (the

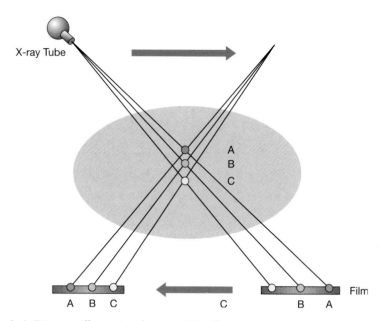

Fig 2-1 Diagram illustrating the principle of tomography.

jaws) is displayed as a flattened out 'panoramic' picture which is created by using slit beam scanning and a form of tomography.

Tomography

Tomography is a technique that uses synchronous movement of an x-ray tube and film cassette carrier, which are linked by a rod that rotates about a pivot point. During the exposure the cassette holder moves in one direction whilst the x-ray tube moves in the opposite direction, as shown in Fig 2-1.

- An object at the pivot point (B) appears at the same place on the film whilst objects above and below this plane have a different linear velocity and so are not sharply shown. Thus objects in plane B are clearly depicted, but objects in other planes, as shown by the letters A and C, are blurred or stretched out and thus not recognisable because they appear in different places on the film.
- The position of the image layer can be adjusted within the object by raising or lowering the pivot point.
- A wide angle of tube and cassette movement results in a narrow zone of sharpness, whilst a small angle of travel in broad zone of sharpness, as illustrated in Fig 2-2.

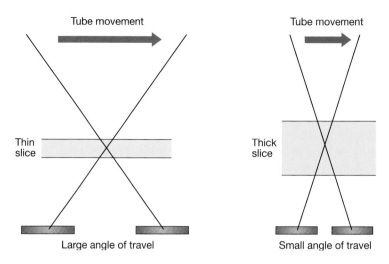

Fig 2-2 Image layer thickness is determined by angle of travel.

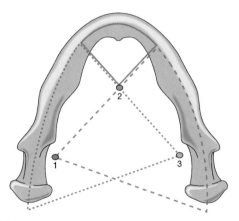

Fig 2-3 Shape of the jaws consisting of the arcs of three circles.

So tomography produces an image of a flat plane, but to record the teeth and jaws it is necessary to image a curved plane that corresponds to the shape of the jaws.

The shape of the jaws can be thought of consisting of the arcs of three circles, as shown in Fig 2-3. The centre or pivot point of each circle is shown by the numbers 1 2 & 3, with their respective arcs. To obtain this curved slice, it is necessary for the tube and cassette carrier to rotate sequentially about these three pivot points. The wide angle employed at the front of the jaws produces a narrow slice.

However, using fixed or stationary centres of rotation results in high radiation doses at the pivot points. This can be overcome by continuously moving or sliding the centres of rotation along a curved path between the three centres, as shown in Fig 2-4.

Slit Beam Imaging

Unlike a conventional dental x-ray set, the panoramic x-ray tube head is designed so that it emits a thin vertical beam of x-rays by incorporating a slit collimator. The x-ray tube is linked to the cassette film holder for synchronous movement. In Fig 2-5, the tube head (A) rotates in a circular horizontal plane around the back of the head and the cassette film holder around the front. As it does so, the slit beam of x-rays scans the jaws and exposes the film sequentially, starting at one end until the whole of the film has been exposed. The cassette holder has a second collimator (B) in front of the cassette to prevent unwanted film exposure. To expose the film, the cassette containing the x-ray film slides passed the secondary collimator, but in the opposite direction to that taken by the direction of travel of the x-ray tube. In this way the jaws are imaged from condyle to condyle (rotational tomography).

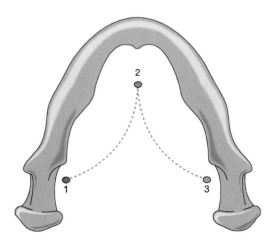

Fig 2-4 Rotation centres sliding from one centre to another.

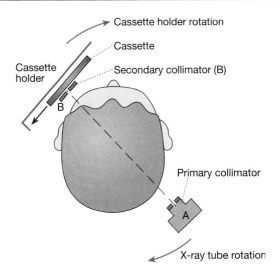

Fig 2-5 Relationship of x-ray tube and cassette holder with primary and beam secondary collimators.

Image Magnification

The centres of rotation act as the 'focus' for the image in the horizontal dimension, whilst the x-ray source (x-ray tube) does so for the vertical dimension. Vertical magnification changes only slightly by altering patient position, but magnification in the horizontal plane varies significantly according to patient position. This is because the magnification in the horizontal plane is determined by the relative speed of rotation of the film and tube in relation to the jaws as they travel around the patient. As a result objects positioned in the selected curved plane show little distortion, but objects either side of this plane will appear either wider or narrower and also less sharp. The image of objects that are placed lateral (labial/buccal) to this plane appear narrow, whilst objects lying medially (lingual/palatal) appear wide, as illustrated in Fig 2-6. Thus, it is important to remember that small changes in patient position greatly affect horizontal magnification. As a consequence, accurate patient positioning is crucial.

Dental Panoramic Technique

All panoramic machines have positioning devices, the commonest being light beam diaphragms (Fig 2-7). Some units use frontal or lateral positioning guides to locate the head (Fig 2-8).

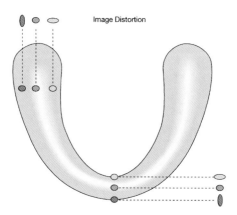

Fig 2-6 Distortion within the image layer. Objects outside the central plane appear distorted, either narrower than normal, if buccally placed or wider when medially placed.

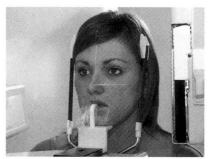

Fig 2-7 Light beams used as a positioning aid.

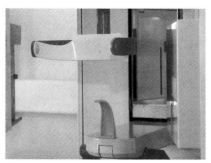

Fig 2-8 Forehead-positioning guide.

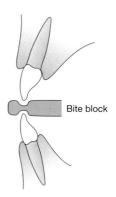

Fig 2-9 Location groove in bite block for central incisors.

The narrowness of the focal trough (the image plane) in the anterior region requires the patient to adopt an edge-to-edge position of the incisor teeth within the bite block (Fig 2-9). This also serves to slightly open the mouth, separating the upper and lower teeth and avoiding superimposition of their crowns.

Practical Procedures

It is essential to read and follow the manufacturer's instructions. However, many machines operate in a similar manner, as described below for a standard DPR.

Preparation

1) Explain the procedure to the patient. Show the bite block groove to indicate that the lower jaw should be slightly opened and protruded forward along the rim of the block to locate the upper and lower incisor teeth into the groove. Briefly outline how the tubehead assembly will rotate around the head and that it is most important to remain stationary during this cycle.
2) Ensure that the patient has removed jewellery, metal dentures, or other radiopaque objects (including chewing gum) that lie in the path of the x-ray beam, and bulky clothing that might interfere with tube and cassette rotation.
3) Cover the bite block with a polythene bag or suitable wrap as an infection control measure (or have sufficient bite blocks to allow sterilisation after each patient).
4) Load the cassette in to the cassette holder, ensuring that the cassette is not back to front or upside down.

Note: The use of a patient lead coat is unnecessary as it offers little or no reduction in patient dose and may intersect the beam, interfering with image formation.

Radiography

1) Invite the patient to place their head into the machine head locator.
2) The height of the tube assembly is adjusted approximately to that of the patient's head height. A useful guide is to ask the patient to stand tall and as straight as possible, and lower the machine until the underneath of the cassette holder is just above shoulder, about the thickness of one's hand. Remember, it is important to adjust the height of the machine to the patient and not vice versa.
3) Ask the patient to place their chin on the chin rest and to bite on to the biteblock so that the central incisors are symmetrically positioned into the

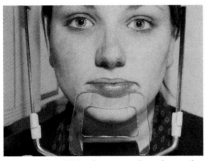

Fig 2-10 Chin locator placed on the anterior aspect of the mandible.

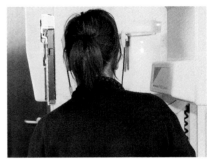

Fig 2-11 The patient's shoulders should be leveled and not as shown here.

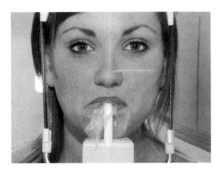

Fig 2-12 Final check that patient is correctly aligned and lips are sealed around bite block.

groove. When the central incisors are missing, the bite block is replaced by the chin locator, which is positioned so that the labial aspect of the mandible is placed against the concave surface of the chin locator, as shown in Fig 2-10.

4) The patient should stand as tall as possible with feet flat on the ground, with their neck and back straight, i.e. in an erect posture. To help the patient remain stable, the patient is instructed to hold on to the patient support handles. Stand behind the patient and check that the shoulders are level. Note that in Fig 2-11, the patient's right shoulder is raised and will interfere with the rotation of the cassette holder .

5) Switch on the light beam diaphragms and gently adjust the patient's head position:
   • laterally, so that the mid-sagittal plane of the face aligns with the central vertical light beam.
   • vertically, so that the horizontal beam delineates the infra-orbital to tra-

gus plane. The occlusal plane will have a slight upward incline from the front to the back of the jaws.

• antero–posteriorly, so that the laterally placed vertical light beam is aligned with either the lateral incisor or canine teeth (this varies according to manufacturer). Fig 2-12 shows a patient's head correctly aligned.

6) Ask the patient to close their lips around the biteblock and place their tongue against the palate in the upper incisor region.

7) Select the correct exposure factors; this will depend on the age and build of the patient. The manufacturer's manual should provide guidance. Local exposure protocols should be to hand for easy reference.

8) 'Prep' the machine and ensure the side head is stabilised with the lateral head supports.

9) Check that the patient has not moved.

10) Remind the patient that the x-ray set will rotate around the head and that they must keep still during the cycle. Retire to a safe position, but observe the patient during the entire exposure.

11) On completion of the exposure, and following infection control guidelines, remove the patient from the machine and retrieve the cassette.

Not all jaws conform to the ideal and accurately fit into the focal trough profile. Some machines have the facility, however, to change the shape of focal trough to accommodate those with a small jaw, such as children, and those who have broad or narrow-shaped jaws.

Many panoramic machines allow the operator to radiograph just selected segments of the jaws. This facility should be considered when only a part of the jaws requires examination, such as assessing wisdom teeth on one side or reviewing a lesion in one quadrant of the jaws.

There are also software programs for specialised projections of the temporomandibular joints, maxillary sinuses and for implant assessment. It is not the purpose of this book to describe these techniques and the reader is referred to the manufacturers' manuals for further details.

Further Reading

Langland OE, Langlais RP, McDavid WD and DelBalso AM. Panoramic Radiology. 2nd Edn. Philadelphia: Lea & Febiger, 1989, Chap. 8, pp 183-223.

Langland OE, Langlais RP and Preece JW. Principles of Dental Imaging. 2nd Edn. Baltimore: Lippincott, Williams & Wilkins, 2002, Chap.9, pp 201-218.

Whaites E. Essentials of Dental Radiography and Radiology. 3rd Edn. Edinburgh: Churchill Livingstone, 2002, Chap. 15, pp 161-176.

White S and Pharoah M. Oral Radiology. 5th Edn. St Louis: Mosby, 2005, Chap. 10, pp 197-198.

Chapter 3
Anatomy

Aim

The aim of this chapter is to outline those anatomical structures that may appear on a DPR. Sectional DPR images are used predominantly throughout this book to clarify the identification of salient features.

Outcome

After studying this chapter the reader should be able to recognize the main anatomical features that appear on dental panoramic radiographs.

Introduction

In order to interpret DPRs, it is essential to be able to recognise normal anatomical features. However, it should be remembered that:
- not every anatomical structure will necessarily appear on each DPR.
- there is variation between individuals
- anatomical features change over time.

There are a large number of anatomical structures that appear on a DPR, so for clarity of presentation, these have been subdivided into:
- hard tissues
- soft tissues
- air shadows
- ghost shadows.

Hard Tissues

It is assumed that those reading this book are familiar with the anatomy of the teeth and so this is not described.

Mandible (Fig 3-1)
A standard DPR shows the whole mandible, although the head of the mandibular condyle is often obscured by superimposition from the skull base.

Sometimes, anatomical features can resemble disease. For example, as shown

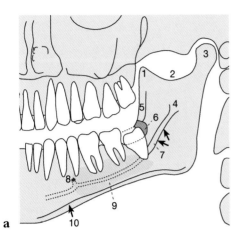

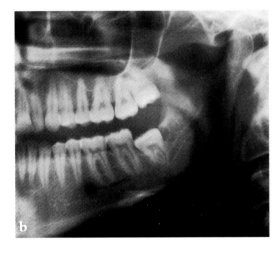

Fig 3-1 a) Diagram of half of the mandible showing the main anatomical features. b) The corresponding half of a DPR.

1. coronoid process
2. sigmoid notch
3. mandibular condyle
4. mandibular foramen
5. external oblique ridge
6. follicular space (around distal aspect of wisdom tooth)
7. inferior alveolar canal (arrows)
8. mental foramen
9. submandibular fossa (coloured pink)
10. cortical margin of the lower border of the mandible (arrowed)

in Fig 3-2, the mental foramen may be superimposed over the apex of the lower second premolar, mimicking a periapical inflammatory lesion. The submandibular fossa can occasionally appear so radiolucent (Fig 3-3) that it may be mistaken for an abnormality, e.g. odontogenic keratocyst.

Maxilla, Antrum, Nasal Skeleton, Zygoma and Temporal Bone
The focal trough passes through only part of the maxilla, maxillary antrum, nasal complex and zygoma. As a consequence, these structures are not fully depicted.

A DPR depicts both maxillary sinuses mainly in lateral profile. Fig 3-4 depicts

Fig 3-2 Mental foramen superimposed over the apex of the lower left second premolar.

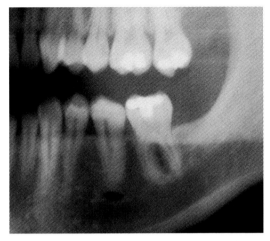

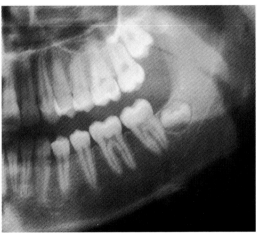

Fig 3-3 Radiolucent submandibular fossa.

the anatomical structures on one side of the upper jaw and associated structures. The floor and posterior walls are well shown and can usually be traced. Some panoramic machines have sinus programmes that place the focal trough in a more favourable position so that more of the maxillary sinuses are depicted.

The maxillary sinuses are rudimentary during the first few years of life, but enlarge during childhood with the formation and eruption of the permanent dentition, to reach full size by adulthood. The floor of the maxillary sinus is often positioned close to the apices of the posterior teeth so that it might appear that roots lie within the antral cavity, but this is not the case the roots

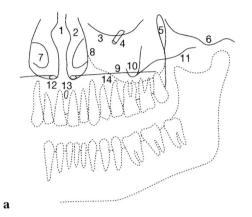

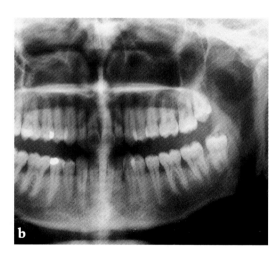

Fig 3-4 a) Diagram of half of the facial skeleton as depicted on a DPR. b) The corresponding half of a DPR.

1. nasal septum
2. nasal airway
3. infra-orbital margin
4. infra-orbital canal
5. pterygomaxillary fissure
6. base of middle cranial fossa
7. inferior turbinate
8. lateral wall of nose/medial wall of maxillary antrum
9. hard palate
10. root of zygoma
11. zygomatic arch
12. floor of maxillary antrum (dotted line)

being superimposed upon the antrum. Following extraction of the upper posterior teeth, the maxillary sinuses slowly enlarge into the alveolus and can, in some circumstances, lie close to the alveolar crest, as shown in Fig 3-5.

Other Bony Structures
These are shown in Fig 3-6.

Soft Tissues

The soft tissues appear as uniform areas of a 'milky' radiopacity that are par-

Fig 3-5 a) Enlargement of the maxillary sinuses following tooth extraction. The sinus floor dips down between the second premolar and second molar teeth to lie close to the alveolar crest. Note the ossified stylohyoid ligament (arrowed). b) In this example the posterior teeth were extracted several years previously. Only a few millimetres separates the maxillary sinus floor from the alveolar crest.

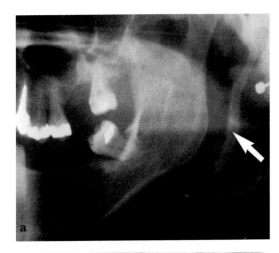

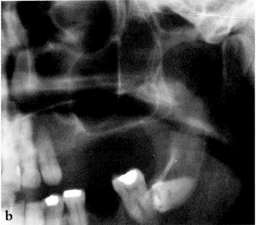

ticularly noticeable when contrasted against radiolucent air shadows. The soft tissues are illustrated in Fig 3-7.

An unusual shadow is the inter-vertebral space between C1 and C2, which is shown in Fig 3-8. This is seen as two sloping radiolucencies that may be superimposed over the apices of the upper central incisor teeth, occasionally resembling periapical disease.

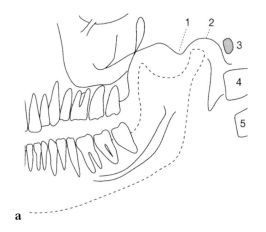

Fig 3-6 a) Diagram of half of a DPR. b) The corresponding half of a DPR.

1. articular eminence
2. glenoid fossa
3. external auditory meatus
4. anterior arch of first cervical vertebra
5. body of second cervical vertebra (arrow)

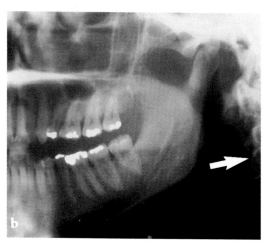

Air Shadows

Air shadows appear radiolucent because of their lack of x-ray photon absorption compared to both the soft and hard tissues. The air shadows are shown in Fig 3-9.

Fig 3-7 a) Diagram showing the soft tissues seen on a DPR. b) Corresponding radiograph showing soft tissue shadows.

1. mucosa covering inferior turbinate
2. soft palate
3. the ear lobe
4. soft tissue of nose
5. dorsum of the tongue
6. outline of lips (visible as a radiolucent shadow as lips are apart)

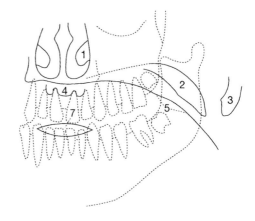

a

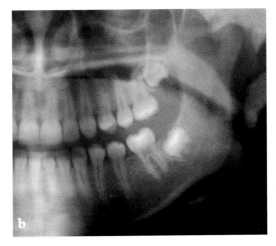

Ghost Shadows

Image formation has been discussed in Chapter 2, where it was shown that a real image is formed when the object lies between the centre of rotation and the x-ray film. However, objects that lie between the x-ray tube head and the centre of rotation may be imaged when they are referred to as 'ghost' images. To create a ghost image the object must be dense and lie posterior

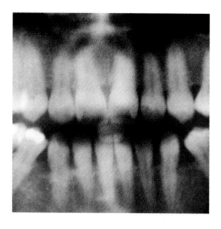

Fig 3-8 Intervertebral spaces between C1 and C2, superimposed upon the apices of the central incisors.

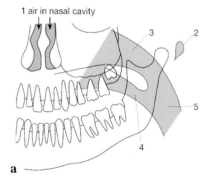

Fig 3-9 a) Diagram showing air shadows seen on a DPR. b) Corresponding radiograph showing air shadows.

1. air in the nasal cavity
2. air in the external auditory meatus
3. air in the nasopharynx;
4. air in oropharynx;
5. air in the common pharynx

Note the hyoid bone (arrowed).

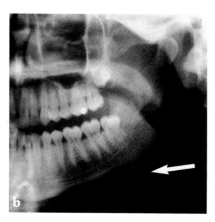

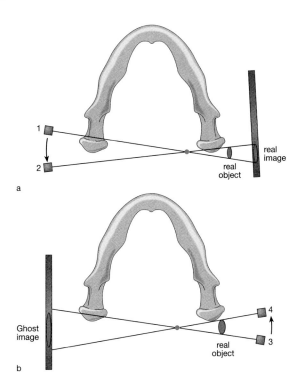

Fig 3-10 Line diagram showing formation of ghost images. Small red circle represents the centre of rotation.

to the centres of rotation. Fig 3-10 illustrates how a ghost image is formed. Examples of ghost shadows include the posterior aspect of the mandible and an ear ring (if not removed), which are projected on to the opposite side of the radiograph. To demonstrate bony ghost shadows, half of a skull was radiographed in a panoramic unit and the resulting images are shown in Fig 3-11a and b.

A ghost image has the following characteristics:
- It appears on the opposite side of the radiograph to its real image counterpart.
- It appears slightly higher up on the radiograph than its real image counterpart, given the approximately 8° upward angulation of the x-ray tube.
- It can be magnified, sometimes markedly so, in the horizontal dimension.
- It will be slightly magnified vertically.

35

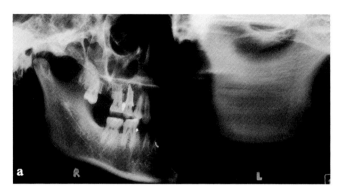

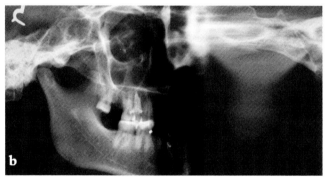

Fig 3-11 Radiographs of half a skull showing ghost images. a) The ghost shadow of the mandible and condyle can be identified on the opposite side to that of the real image. b) This radiograph was taken with the skull placed more anteriorly, which has resulted in greatly reduced ghost shadowing of the mandible, with just the "ghost" condylar head remaining visible.

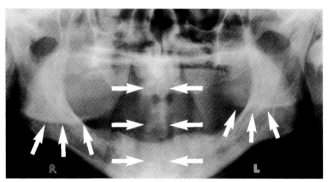

Fig 3-12 DPR showing ghost shadows of the mandible (vertical arrows indicating their lower limit) and of the cervical vertebrae (horizontal arrows). Both appear as radiopaque shadows.

The following structures may appear as ghost images:
- Posterior body and angle of the mandible. This is seen as a broad radiopaque area (arrows) in Fig 3-12.
- Cervical vertebrae. This appears as a blurred vertical (column like) radiopacity in the middle lower half of the radiograph (Fig 3-12).
- Earrings (see also chapter 6).

Further Reading

Langland OE, Langlais RP, McDavid WD and DelBalso AM. Panoramic Radiology. 2nd Edn. Philadelphia: Lea & Febiger, 1989, Chap. 8, pp 183-223.

Langland OE, Langlais RP and Preece JW . Principles of Dental Imaging. 2nd Edn. Baltimore: Lippincott, Williams & Wilkins, 2002, Chap. 9, pp 201-218.

Chapter 4
Radiation Dose and Risk in Panoramic Radiography

Aim

The aims of this chapter are to provide the practitioner with the principles of how radiation damage occurs, to describe the concepts of radiation dose and risk, to discuss the level of dose delivered and the physical methods of dose reduction achievable in panoramic radiography.

Outcome

After studying this chapter, the reader should understand the biological effects of ionising radiation, the relevance and the method of computation of effective dose and risk and should also be conversant with the various methods to reduce dose to patients when using panoramic radiography.

Introduction

Following Roentgen's discovery of x-rays at the end of the 19th century, medical and dental practitioners were not slow to see the potential diagnostic benefits of an x-ray examination. They also became rapidly aware of the damaging effects of x-rays to both themselves and their patients.

The Biological Effects of Panoramic Radiography

During a radiographic examination, millions of x-ray photons pass through the region of the body under review. X-ray photons have the potential to cause damage by a process known as ionisation. In this process, one or more electrons are removed from atoms, and also the bonds between the atoms themselves are often disrupted. Although damage can occur anywhere within the cell itself, damage affecting the DNA in the chromosomes is the most critical. DNA does have the potential to repair itself, but this is dependent on the degree of damage sustained (Fig 4-1). If repair is impossible, the damaged portion of the DNA of the chromosome remains permanently altered as a mutation. The period between exposure to x-rays and the clinical diagnosis of a tumour is generally many years.

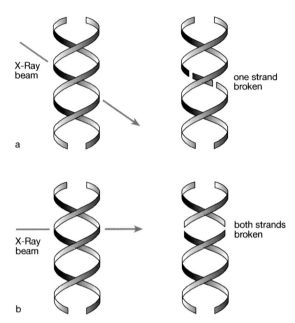

Fig 4-1 DNA damage caused by irradiation. a) Single strand breaks can be repaired using the complementary strand as a template. b) Other damage may be irreparable and have serious long-lasting effects.

A detailed knowledge of the dose received from any radiographic examination allows a scientific estimation of the possible risk of tumour induction for the patient. There is evidence to show that exposure to dental radiographic examinations can result in an increased risk of brain, salivary gland and thyroid tumours. These effects are random and have no threshold radiation dose below which they will not occur. These occurrences are referred to as 'chance' or stochastic effects, in which the magnitude of the risk is proportional to the radiation dose.

Radiation Units

Measurement of Dose
The dose delivered to the patient can be measured in several ways. One of the easiest ways is to place dosemeters on the patient's skin to record entrance dose, and the resultant measurement is recorded in milligrays (mGy). A more meaningful measurement of dose is to carry out a calculation of effective dose. The calculation of effective dose requires detailed knowledge of indi-

vidual doses to specific organs. Each of these specific organs has an individual weighting factor based on the contribution of that organ to the total overall risk of developing a fatal tumour/nonfatal tumour or promoting a severe hereditary effect in the progeny.

Effective dose expresses the multiplicity of doses affecting the variety of tissue types and organs encountered as the x-ray beam traverses the patient. These are then represented as a single value of 'whole body' detriment. The theoretical calculation relies upon either laboratory studies or computer modelling, and the derived figure can subsequently be used to estimate radiation risk. Effective dose is measured in units of energy absorption per unit mass (Joules/kg) called the Sievert. For dental exposures, in which doses are relatively low, the measurement is recorded in microsieverts (µSv) representing one millionth of a Sievert.

Effective Dose and Risk in Panoramic Radiography
Using recently published research on panoramic radiography, the effective dose for panoramic radiography ranges from 3.85 µSv to 30 µSv. The corresponding risk of fatal cancer per million ranges from 0.21 to 1.9, respectively. The rates quoted for risk relate to an adult patient of 30 years of age. Risk is age-dependent, being highest for the young and lowest for the elderly. The modifying multiplication factors used to account for age in risk estimation are given in Table 4-1.

Table 4-1 **Risk in relation to age** (Based upon ICRP Publication 60. *Radiation Protection. 1990 recommendations of the International Commission on Radiological Protection.* Annals of the ICRP 21).

Age group (years)	Multiplicative factor for risk
<10	x 3
10-20	x 2
20-30	x 1.5
30-50	x 0.5
50-80	x 0.3
80+	Negligible risk

The variability seen in the calculation of effective dose and risk is a reflection of the many variables involved in producing a DPR and also relates to the method of dose computation. The latter problem centres on whether the dose to the salivary glands should be given a special weighting in the calculation of effective dose. Salivary gland tissue, in particular the parotid gland, receives the highest dose in the head and neck region during any panoramic exposure. As salivary gland tissue has been shown to be radiosensitive, it seems likely that any computation of effective dose without inclusion of salivary tissue must represent a severe underestimation.

In the United Kingdom, older panoramic equipment is commonly found in use within general practice. Generally, higher levels of dose and consequently risk occurs when using equipment of this type. This was substantiated by a recent study that examined 12% of UK panoramic equipment; the highest and the lowest dose recorded differed by a factor of 200.

How Can We Reduce Dose to Our Patients?

Newer panoramic units tend to include several dose-reducing features, including the use of:
- constant potential ('direct current') x-ray generation
- field limitation techniques
- rare-earth screens
- digital technology.

Constant Potential ('direct current') X-Ray Generation

The typical x-ray unit uses a system known as half-wave rectification to produce the x-ray beam. The changing polarity of the alternating current (AC) gives rise to a pulsed output only during the positive half of the cycle. During this period, the voltage across the tube fluctuates from zero to its maximum level. The resultant x-ray beam therefore consists of both low and high-energy photons, with the former serving little purpose but to increase patient dose.

To overcome the above problems, x-ray equipment has been developed that ensures a constant potential across the x-ray tube. The effect is accomplished by either capacitor smoothing, triodes for ripple suppression, or a three-phase supply. The resultant x-ray beam has a higher proportion of high energy photons than those produced by conventional equipment operating at the same kilovoltage. The use of constant potential equip-

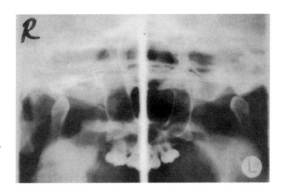

Fig 4-2 Segmental DPRs of the left and right temporo-mandibular joints.

ment allows the clinician to produce radiographs of adequate density and contrast while using a shorter exposure time, thereby reducing dose to the patient.

Field Limitation Techniques

Field limitation techniques allow the operator to selectively image certain structures, such as the temporomandibular region (Fig 4-2), the maxillary sinuses, and the third molar region, and also to modify coverage according to patient type, i.e., either for a child or an adult. Field limitation techniques produce significant dose reduction for the patient.

The Use of Rare-Earth Screens

Dose reduction is achieved by employing rare-earth screens. These materials are efficient in absorbing a higher proportion (60%) of x-ray photons reaching the cassette than the traditional calcium tungstate screen. Rare-earth materials are also more efficient in converting x-ray photons into visible light again when compared with the calcium tungstate screens. Therefore, exposure factors can be adjusted in the light of the increased efficiency of the rare-earth screen.

Digital Panoramic Systems

Manufacturers of panoramic equipment have adopted digital technology using either a charge-coupled device or photostimulable phosphors. These systems have been reported to reduce dose by allowing images to be acquired at lower exposures while maintaining the full grey-scale of conventional radiographs using image enhancement techniques.

The Risks Associated with Panoramic Radiography

Everything we do in life is associated with risk, but various occupations and particular types of activity can result in an unacceptable level of risk to the individual. Examples of these activities are deep-sea fishing with a fatal accident rate of one in 1,000 and rock climbing for 2.5 hours which carries a one in 10,000 risk of death.

The annual exposure of the UK population from all sources of ionising radiation during 1999 is shown in Table 4-2. Medical radiation comprises the largest man-made component of radiation exposure to the population, representing 14% of the total overall annual dose. During the past 30 years, the number of UK dental radiographic examinations has increased by 50% compared with a 5% rise in hospital radiographic examinations over the same period. Categorising this increase by dental film type reveals that DPRs have increased by 181% compared to a 25% rise for intraoral radiography.

Should we be worried about risks when carrying out radiographic examinations on our patients? The risk of cancer following any radiation exposure has been derived from studies of three groups of individuals:
• survivors of the atomic bombs at Nagasaki and Hiroshima
• populations exposed for medical reasons
• individuals exposed occupationally.

Using the extrapolated data derived from these groups, it is possible to derive risk models. It should be remembered that risk is age-dependent and is therefore quantifiable (Table 4-1).

The dose given for any radiographic examination is dependent on the age of the patient, the type of examination undertaken and the techniques used to produce the final image. The effective dose and risk for a variety of radiographic examinations are given in Table 4-3. Practitioners often ask for a comparison in dose and risk between different examinations. Such a question is almost impossible to answer definitively because of the large number of permutations of equipment variables for both panoramic and intraoral examinations. Consideration must also be given to the age of the patient under investigation. It is possible, therefore, for one practice to be using equipment where the dose for panoramic radiography greatly exceeds that for the total number of intraoral films needed to give the same clinical information, while in another practice the reverse may be true.

Table 4-2 **Annual exposure of the UK population from all sources of ionising radiation** (Based upon: Hughes JS. Ionising Radiation Exposure of the UK population: 1999 review. 2001, Chilton, NRPB-R311.)

Source	Average annual dose (μSv)	Approximate percentage of total
Natural		
Cosmic	320	12%
Gamma	350	13.5%
Internal	270	10%
Radon	1300	50%
Artificial		
Medical	370	14%
Occupational	6	0.2%
Fallout	4	0.2%
Disposals	0.3	<0.1%
Consumer products	0.1	<0.1%
Total (rounded)	2,600	100%

Table 4-3 **Effective dose and risk to adult patients for a range of radiographic examinations to the head and neck region** (Based upon: 1. National Radiological Protection Board. Guidelines on patient dose to promote the optimisation of protection for diagnostic medical exposures. Vol. 10. No 1. Chilton: National Radiological Protection Board,1999. 2. Faculty of General Dental Practitioners (UK). Selection Criteria for Dental Radiography. 2nd edition. Eds: Pendlebury ME, Horner K, Eaton KA., Royal College of Surgeons of England, London, 2004.)

Radiographic examination	Effective dose (μSv)	Estimated risk of cancer (per million)
CT head	2000	100★
PA skull	30	1.49★
CT maxilla	100 - 3324	8 - 242[+]
CT mandible	364 - 1202	18.2 - 88[+]
Radionuclide examination of bone (99mTc)	4000	200★
Panoramic radiograph	3.85 - 30	0.21 - 1.9[+]
Intraoral radiograph	1- 8.3	0.02 - 0.6[+]

★Approximate lifetime risk for patients aged 16-69 years: multiply by two for paediatric patients and divide by five for geriatric patients.

[+]Approximate lifetime risk for patients aged 30 years: use the multiplication factors given in Table 4.2 according to patient age.

Conclusion

Risk is associated with everything we do in life, and having a radiographic examination is no exception. Although the risk in dental panoramic radiography is small, UK practitioners have a legislative responsibility to reduce dose to their patients. While not all practitioners will have access to 'state-of-the-art' panoramic equipment and may not wish or be able to invest in new equipment, the simple expedient of changing to rare-earth screens would result in a significant dose reduction.

Further Reading

Whaites E. Essentials of Dental Radiography and Radiology. 3rd Edn. Edinburgh: Churchill Livingstone, 2002.

White SC and Pharoah MJ. Oral Radiology 5th Edn. St. Louis: Mosby 2004.

Chapter 5
The Use of Panoramic Radiography in General Dental Practice

Aim

The aims of this chapter are to give the practitioner an insight into the principles of radiographic justification, the limiting factors of panoramic radiography, and to discuss the uses of panoramic radiography in clinical practice.

Outcome

After studying this chapter, the reader should understand the limitations of the panoramic radiograph as well as its diagnostic accuracy. Those areas of clinical practice in which scientific evidence supports the use of panoramic radiography should also be recognised.

Introduction

Although x-rays have become an accepted part of everyday clinical practice, each radiographic examination poses a potential risk to the patient. This is true for all medical exposures, even for those that deliver lower doses, as is typically the case in dental radiography.

Every x-ray examination should produce a net benefit for the patient by adding new information to help in their management. This principle of weighing the potential diagnostic benefits of a radiographic examination against the possible individual detriment is a well-established tenet of radiation protection.

The process of justifying an appropriate radiographic examination follows on from a careful history and a thorough clinical examination of the patient. The practice of 'routine' or 'screening' radiography cannot be sanctioned, as such examinations are carried out irrespective of the presence or absence of clinical signs and symptoms. Consideration must also be given to the prevalence of the disease, its rate of progression and, most importantly, the diagnostic efficacy of the radiographic technique chosen to image the suspected pathology.

The Development of Clinical Guidelines

The development of clinical guidelines has simplified the process of selecting radiographs for a particular clinical situation. Such guidelines are often referred to as 'referral criteria' or 'selection criteria' and have been developed for both medical and dental radiography. The development of guidelines involves a rigorous and robust evaluation of all the available scientific evidence and encompasses an extensive literature review using explicit methodologies.

Radiographic Referral Criteria have been defined as 'descriptions of clinical conditions derived from patient signs, symptoms and history that identify patients who are likely to benefit from a particular radiographic technique' (Dental Radiography Patient Selection Criteria Panel and Joseph LP, 1987). As with any guidelines, these are not intended to be rigid constraints on clinical practice, but a concept of good practice against which the needs of the individual patient can be considered.

The Limitations of the Panoramic Image

Every radiographic examination has its limitations and can never be seen as a totally accurate representation. Magnification and an unsharp image will undoubtedly affect radiographic accuracy, while the type of image receptor used has an impact upon the ability to see fine detail. Resolution is the term used to describe the ability of the image receptor to differentiate structures that lie close together. Resolution is objectively measured by radiographing test objects containing very fine metal wires of decreasing thickness and intervening distance. It can be expressed as the number of line pairs per millimetre (l.p. mm^{-1}).

Dental intraoral film has an extremely high resolution of around 20 l.p. mm^{-1}. Any radiographic technique, such as panoramic radiography, that relies upon intensifying screens to form the final image is inevitably associated with some loss of information when compared with conventional direct intraoral film (Fig 5-1). Most intensifying screen/film cassette combinations have a resolution of around 5 to 6 l.p. mm^{-1} (Fig 5-1).

Other factors, such as the setting of incorrect exposure factors and poor processing, can further affect the resultant optical density and contrast of the final image (see Chapter 6).

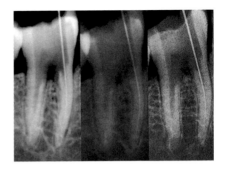

Fig 5-1 Three radiographs of the same tooth taken using conventional dental film (right), an intensifying screen/ film cassette combination (centre), and a digital intraoral x-ray system (left). Conventional dental film displays superior image sharpness.

In panoramic radiography, other factors that are directly attributable to the technique itself can further reduce resolution. These include:

- magnification variations within the image
- the overlap of posterior teeth
- the superimposition of soft tissue and secondary shadows.

Magnification Variations

DPRs have a complex pattern of magnification as a direct result of the mechanics of image production. To obtain an ideal DPR, the operator must ensure that the patient is correctly positioned in the centre of the image plane. The image plane is also often referred to as the focal trough.

Most modern types of equipment have devices, such as positioning lights, bite blocks, chin rests and lateral side guides, to ensure that the patient is correctly positioned. Within the focal trough, both horizontal and vertical magnification are equally matched. If the patient is inaccurately positioned, a discrepancy between the vertical and horizontal magnification of teeth and jaws occurs. These inaccuracies are usually most marked in the anterior region of the jaws (see Chapter 6).

Overlap of Adjacent Teeth

The ideal projection geometry of the panoramic x-ray beam is perpendicular to the dental arch throughout its rotational movement around the patient's head. This ideal has proved difficult to achieve, in particular for the premolar/molar region, and results in a variable amount of overlap of tooth contact points. Newer equipment has incorporated innovative projectional geometry in an attempt to overcome the problem, but this has not signifi-

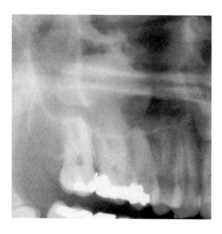

Fig 5-2 Part of a DPR displaying overlap of tooth contact points in the premolar region. Note the antral mucous retention cyst above the molar teeth.

cantly improved the detection of approximal caries in the premolar region (Fig 5-2).

Superimpositions

Panoramic images are further degraded, to a variable degree, by shadows of soft tissues and surrounding air (Fig 5-3). Secondary images of the spine and mandible (Fig 5-4) further reduce diagnostic quality. These images can be reduced by careful positioning of the patient.

Diagnostic Accuracy and Efficacy of Panoramic Radiography

Radiographs are an accepted part of clinical practice, but it is important to remember that every x-ray examination has a limit to its degree of accuracy in diagnosing pathology.

How do we Assess Radiographic Accuracy?

Obviously, the aim of any diagnostic test is to identify a particular disease occurring in an apparently healthy population. Whenever any diagnostic test is developed, it must always be compared with the true diagnosis in order to measure its effectiveness. To assess effectiveness we need to employ two statistical indices:

- sensitivity
- specificity.

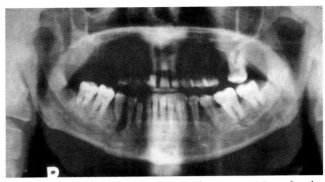

Fig 5-3 DPR displaying a pronounced air shadow above the tongue. Note also the mandibular fracture in the right premolar region.

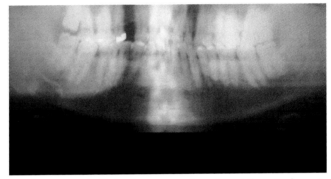

Fig 5-4 Patient is placed asymmetrically in the panoramic unit and there is also evidence of slumping rather than an upright position. This has resulted in severe secondary shadowing of the posterior parts of the mandible and the cervical spine. An incidental finding is a Stafne's bone cavity evident just above the lower cortex at the right angle of the mandible.

Sensitivity determines how good the test is at finding those with the disease, i.e., the proportion of disease positives who test positive. On the other hand, specificity shows how good the test is at excluding those without the disease, i.e., the proportion of disease negatives that are test negatives.

It is probably easier to relate these statistical indices to everyday clinical practice, such as caries identification. Therefore, sensitivity records the 'true positive' fraction of caries lesions in the oral cavity and expresses them as a percentage. Specificity is the proportion of healthy tooth surfaces that would be correctly identified by the diagnostic test, i.e., the 'true negative' fraction. Obviously, the perfect diagnostic system would have 100% sensitivity and

100% specificity. Sensitivities less than 100% indicate that there will be a proportion of undetected pathology ('false negative' diagnoses), i.e., the test identifies the tooth surface as having no caries involvement when, in fact, it has decay. Similarly, specificities less than 100% indicate that there would be a proportion of undetected healthy sites misdiagnosed as diseased ('false positive' diagnoses). It is only by understanding these terms that one can quantify the diagnostic validity of different imaging techniques.

The Diagnostic Value of Panoramic Radiography for Common Dental Pathosis

Caries Diagnosis

Sensitivity values for caries diagnosis using panoramic radiography are much lower than those recorded using bitewing radiographs (Fig 5-5). Panoramic radiographic sensitivity values for approximal caries vary considerably in different regions of the oral cavity. This variation ranges from 8% in the incisor region to 30% in the premolar region, with the highest sensitivity values (52%) occurring in the molar region. The overall sensitivity levels for approximal caries diagnosis using panoramic equipment varies between studies and ranges from 22% to 37%. In addition, the panoramic technique also produces a high level of false negative readings of 80% in the premolar region.

By contrast, bitewing radiography shows much higher values of sensitivity and specificity for approximal caries. One systematic review of bitewing radiography reported figures of 66% and 95% for sensitivity and specificity, respectively, for the cavitated dentinal lesion.

Periodontal Disease

The diagnosis of periodontal disease is dependent upon a thorough clinical examination of the patient. Both intraoral and panoramic radiography have limitations when assessing periodontal bone loss. Both intraoral and extraoral radiographic techniques tend to underestimate bone loss, with reported figures ranging from 13 to 32% for panoramic radiography to 11 to 23% for bitewing radiography, and between 9 and 20% for periapical radiography.

In panoramic radiography, the degree of inaccuracy is further compounded by the upward 8-degree angulation of the beam. This results in an underestimation of bone loss in the mandible and, conversely, an overestimation of bone loss in the maxilla. In addition, difficulties may well be encountered

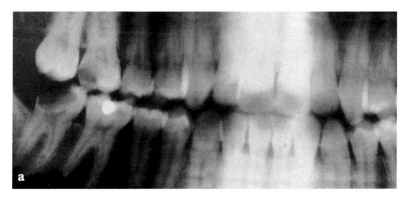

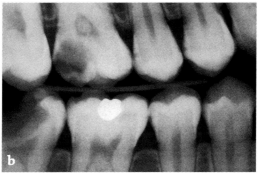

Fig 5-5 The improved sensitivity for caries lesions of intraoral bitewing radiography b) compared with the DPR a) is shown. Overlap on the upper right premolars on the DPR has obscured approximal lesions. Note also the 'false positive' radiolucent lesion mesially on the lower right first premolar produced by the air shadow of the commisure of the mouth on the DPR.

in accurately identifying the periodontal bone margin (Fig 5-6), especially in the anterior and premolar regions of the jaws.

Effective imaging of complex bone loss, such as furcation involvement and vertical defects, is challenging for both periapical and panoramic radiography. Complex lesions such as these are more adequately imaged using bitewing radiographs, which have the advantage that they may have been taken for caries assessment.

Periapical Inflammatory Pathology
Intraoral periapical radiography is recognised as being superior to panoramic radiography in the detection of periapical inflammatory pathology. Again,

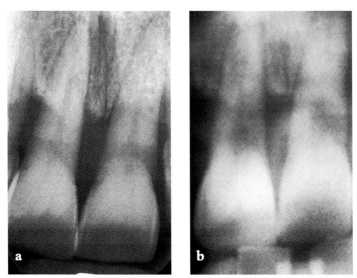

Fig 5-6 The improved resolution of intraoral film a) compared with the DPR b) is depicted. The DPR has been cut down to show only the area of interest.

sensitivity levels vary depending on the study type and the region of the oral cavity examined. DPRs give extremely low sensitivity values of 29% in the mandibular incisor/canine region. By contrast, sensitivity levels of 65% have been calculated when assessing periapical disease using periapical radiography.

The Diagnostic Value of Panoramic Radiography for Other Pathology

In this section, an assessment is made of the efficacy of the DPR in diagnosing less frequently occurring pathology.

Prior to Oral Surgery

In the United Kingdom, clinicians are expected to follow strict guidelines to assess whether third molars require removal. These guidelines stress that wisdom teeth should not be removed unless there is a valid clinical reason for doing so, such as repeated episodes of pericoronitis or unrestorable dental decay. The DPR gives important information for the assessment of third molars prior to their surgical removal (Fig 5-7). In the case of third mandibular molars, this assessment includes the distance to the lower border of the mandible and the course and the relationship of the inferior dental canal relative to the tooth. The latter assessment may well require a supplemental

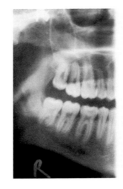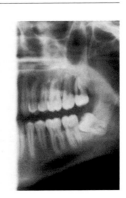

Fig 5-7 DPR showing an impacted third molar and its relationship to the inferior dental canal and the lower cortex.

periapical view of the third molar. It is important to remember that radiography is needed only when clinical guidelines for removal have been met and surgical removal is imminent.

In general practice, the remainder of surgical treatment encompasses the removal of retained roots, apicectomy and the enucleation of small cysts. In the majority of patients, the area under consideration can often be adequately imaged using intraoral radiography alone.

The routine use of preoperative radiography prior to a simple extraction is not supported by the literature. Obviously, this would not be the case in those patients with an impacted or buried tooth or when managing retained roots. If, however, the clinical history and examination reveal compelling evidence to support a preoperative radiograph, then a periapical radiograph is the obvious choice. Before embarking on a radiographic examination, it is always right to check the patient's clinical records for previous films of the region, as these may be sufficient.

The Detection of Facial Fractures
Panoramic radiography has been shown to be very effective in diagnosing mandibular fractures in the symphyseal, parasymphseal, body and angle regions. Fractures affecting the high condylar neck region are difficult to diagnose when using panoramic radiography alone, and similarly, the technique has a limited ability to detect mid-facial fractures. Various studies have shown, however, that poor patient positioning and processing can dramatically reduce diagnostic yield (Fig 5-8).

It can be argued that if there is clinical evidence of a bony facial fracture, it

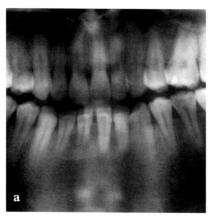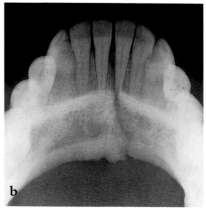

Fig 5-8 Poor positioning of the patient obscures the midline fracture on the DPR a) but it is obvious on the lower oblique occlusal view b).

is probably best for the dentist to refer the patient for a complete radiographic examination at the hospital where treatment will be performed.

Sinus Disease
DPRs have limitations when evaluating antral sinus pathology, such as mucosal thickening, bony changes and malignancy. As with facial fractures, it is probably best to refer patients for specialist opinion in a hospital environment where appropriate imaging can be performed.

Identification of Systemic Disease
DPRs have been recommended as a method of identifying certain systemic diseases, including vascular disease and osteoporosis.

DPRs have been reported to be very effective in alerting the dentist to the presence of calcified carotid arterial plaques. Unfortunately, many of the published studies have been performed without validation of the findings or a measurement of the benefit to the patient of the identification of these lesions. More importantly, justification of a DPR for this purpose cannot be supported when the 'nonradiographic' alternative technique of a duplex ultrasound examination would give much more meaningful information for the future management of the patient.

In osteoporotic patients (Fig 5-9), the measurements of specific sites in the mandible, as located on a DPR, allow an assessment of the degree of min-

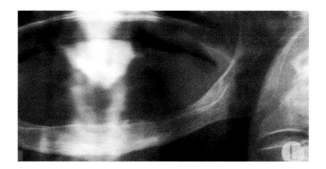

Fig 5-9 DPR of an osteoporotic patient showing pronounced thinning of cortical boundaries (i.e., the lower cortex).

eralised bone loss. The results show a modest diagnostic accuracy compared with other more established methods of diagnosing low bone mineral density. Problems have been encountered, however, in obtaining consistency in measurements amongst observers. Consequently, the practical potential of DPTs for identifying patients at risk of osteoporosis in a primary care setting remains uncertain.

The Assessment of Temporomandibular Joint Pathology
The majority of patients presenting with pain in the temporomandibular region tend to be suffering from soft tissue conditions such as myofascial pain-dysfunction or an internal joint derangement. In the former condition, there are no related bony abnormalities of the joints, while in the latter, bony changes (sclerosis, erosions, osteophytes, and flattening) are seen infrequently, usually in association with nonreducing and perforated discs.

As such, the clinician must consider the usefulness and appropriateness of panoramic radiography in assessing the temporomandibular region in the light of these findings. Even in the minority of patients with a bony abnormality, it is doubtful whether the findings of any plain radiographic examination will influence initial management, particularly in a primary care setting. Recent research has confirmed that in the majority of patients with temporomandibular disorders, panoramic radiography did not provide any information that influenced the diagnosis or patient management.

The limitations of panoramic radiography in the temporomandibular joint (TMJ) region must also be considered. Changes in bony structures can generally only be made on the lateral slope and central parts of the condyle, given the oblique orientation of the beam relative to the long axis of the condyle. In addition, only gross changes involving the articular eminence and glenoid

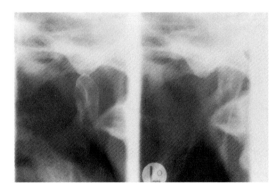

Fig 5-10 This sectional DPR shows (on the right of the image) the position of the condyle in the 'normal' position, obscured by overlying bone. The image on the left shows the same patient with the mouth open to clear this superimposition.

fossa are evident due to superimposition by the base of the skull and zygomatic arch (Fig 5-10).

A recent consultative document reviewed those conditions affecting the TMJ in order to develop guidelines as to which conditions would benefit from imaging. The following fell into this category:

• trauma involving the TMJ
• significant dysfunction or alteration in the range of motion of the joint
• sensory or motor alterations in the TMJ region
• significant changes in occlusion (i.e. anterior open bite, posterior open bite, and mandibular shift).

There was also consensus agreement that imaging should not be considered in those patients who present with no other signs or symptoms except joint sounds. Obviously, clinical studies will be required to evaluate how effective these criteria would be in reducing unnecessary imaging of the temporomandibular joint.

Conclusions

The balance of the available evidence suggests that DPRs are less effective for the diagnosis of common dental pathoses (dental caries, periodontal bone loss, and periapical inflammatory disease) than intraoral radiographs. As far as other diagnostic uses are concerned, DPRs are extremely useful in the assessment of impacted third molars prior to their surgical removal. They have also been shown to be extremely effective in the assessment of mandibular fractures, provided that the patient is correctly positioned and the film adequately processed. They are valuable in the assessment of lesions too large

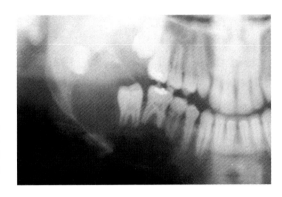

Fig 5-11 DPR of a large ameloblastoma showing expansion of the mandibular body. There is also extensive root resorption.

to be visualised on intra-oral radiographs or in regions not covered by intra-oral films.

Routine Screening by Panoramic Radiography

In several clinical specialties and amongst certain categories of patients, panoramic radiography screening has been reported to have become commonplace. These patient groups and clinical specialties include:
• new adult patients
• edentulous patients
• orthodontics
• implant therapy.

Panoramic Radiography for the New Adult Patient

The routine practice of supplementing the clinical examination of a new adult patient by a 'screening' DPR is well established. It has been shown that such screening examinations mirror the natural prevalence of disease in the jaws, whilst achieving little except the diagnosis of a limited number of insignificant anomalies. More importantly, the percentage of patients receiving any benefit from 'screening' examinations is extremely low and the pathology found is often non-urgent. In fact, a thorough clinical examination would have been sufficient in many cases to alert the clinician to the possibility of the presence of pathology.

The practice of 'screening' is defended on the basis of the possibility of detecting large cysts and tumours. This argument ignores the low prevalence of such lesions and the fact that pathology of this type often has signs or symptoms that would indicate radiography (Fig 5-11).

Research has shown that a DPR may well be appropriate in those patients who present with a grossly neglected mouth. In these patients, there are significant numbers of clinically determined caries lesions and periapical pathology along with established periodontal disease. In such cases, the DPR can rapidly identify teeth of poor prognosis and those that require a more detailed intraoral radiographic examination.

Edentulous Patients

An edentulous patient attending without any clinical signs or symptoms does not require a radiographic examination. If the clinical examination identifies limited pathology, such as a retained root, then an intraoral radiograph is the most appropriate radiographic examination. For more advanced forms of treatment, such as multiple implant placement, more advanced imaging (i.e. cross-sectional imaging) may be the most appropriate.

Panoramic Radiography within Orthodontic Practice

In orthodontic practice, the technique of screening with panoramic radiography is commonplace. This is suprising, as research has shown that, in a majority of patients, a clinical examination supplemented by study models is often sufficient to derive a correct treatment plan.

More worryingly, orthodontic radiographs appear to have a limited role in altering the clinician's final diagnosis, with between 16% and 37% of radiographs effecting a change[2-5]. For treatment planning, the need for orthodontic radiography becomes even more tenuous, with only 4% to 20% of films resulting in altered treatment[2-5].

The use of clinical indicators and algorithms has been effective in correctly assessing those children in need of orthodontic treatment. As a by-product of these methods, there is a dramatic reduction in the numbers of orthodontic films needed, and this occurs without compromising patient care.

While such research does not provide evidence that panoramic radiography is unnecessary for orthodontic treatment, it raises the question as to whether its present use is excessive.

Panoramic Radiography in Implantology

Imaging is obviously essential in implantology to provide information for treatment planning, the quantity and quality of bone in the proposed implant sites, and postoperatively to assess implant osteointegration, bone healing, and to review the fixture.

Although the film can image all of the jaws, certain disadvantages must be taken into consideration. These include:

- high inherent magnification (20-30%)
- geometric distortion both vertically and horizontally
- lingually positioned objects (such as inferior alveolar canal) cast superiorly, thereby reducing accuracy
- technical errors due to incorrect patient position, reducing measurement accuracy
- no buccolingual measurement possible
- reduced resolution
- effective localisation of anatomy may be difficult

Dimensional accuracy is of paramount importance in implant placement. When using panoramic radiography, care must be taken as bone height measurements can deviate from their true value. Therefore, alternative methods of imaging should be employed if the clinical case dictates precision.

Conclusions

There is sufficient clear evidence from the literature to support a radical reassessment of the usefulness of panoramic radiography in all aspects of dental practice. Although panoramic radiography does undoubtedly have a role to play in clinical practice (Table 5-1), this will probably be much more accurately focussed when using an evidenced-based approach as outlined in this chapter. Individual values and judgements on any radiographic technique are often coloured by nonclinical factors. The movement towards evidence-based practice eliminates the influence of such nonclinical aspects of dental care by using techniques that concentrate upon clinical efficacy.

Before any imaging is considered for a patient, it is important that the clinician asks certain questions:

- Which imaging technique will have the greatest diagnostic accuracy and highest precision?
- Will the use of the imaging technique affect the clinical management?
- Is the use of the imaging technique likely to improve the clinical outcome?

This chapter will have given the practitioner the information with which to answer these questions, thereby ensuring that the patient receives the maximum diagnostic yield from their radiographic examination.

Table 5-1 **Suggested selection criteria for panoramic radiography** (Based upon: Selection Criteria for Dental Radiography. Faculty of General Dental Practitioners, Royal College of Surgeons of England, London, 2004.)

Where a bony lesion or unerupted tooth is of a size or position that precludes its complete demonstration on intraoral radiographs.

A grossly neglected mouth with significant numbers of clinically determined caries lesions and periapical pathology along with established periodontal disease (other than simple gingivitis) and where there is pocketing greater than 6 mm in depth.

For the assessment of wisdom teeth prior to planned surgical intervention. Routine radiography of unerupted third molars is not recommended.

As part of an orthodontic assessment where there is a clinical need to know the state of the dentition and the presence/absence of teeth. The use of clinical criteria to select patients rather than to routinely screen patients is essential.

Reference

1. Dental Radiographic Patient Selection Criteria Panel and Joseph L P (1987). The Selection of Patients for X-ray Examinations. Rockville, Maryland: Department of Health and Human Services, Public Health Service, Food and Drug Administration, Center for Devices and Radiological Health, HHS Publication FDA 88-8273.

2. Bruks A, Enberg K, Nordqvist I, Hansson AS, Jansson L, Svenson B. Radiographic examinations as an aid to orthodontic diagnosis and treatment planning. Swed Dent J 1999; 23: 77-85.

3. Han UK, Vig KWL, Weintraud JA, Vig PS, Kowalski CJ. Consistency of orthodontic treatment decisions relative to diagnostic records. Am J Orthop Dentofac Orthop 1991; 100: 212-219.

4. Atchinson KA, Luke LS, White SC. Contribution of pretreatment radiographs to orthodontists' decision making. Oral Surg Oral Med Oral Pathol 1991; 71: 238-245.

5. Atchinson KA, Luke LS, White SC. An algorithm for ordering pretreatment orthodontic radiographs. Am J Orthod Dentofac Orthop 1992: 102:29-44

Further Reading

British Orthodontic Society. Guidelines for the use of radiographs in clinical orthodontics. Isaacson KG and Thom AR, eds. 2nd edn. London: British Orthodontic Society, 2001.

National Institute for Clinical Excellence. Technology Appraisals Guidance- No. 1. Guidance on the removal of wisdom teeth. 2000. National Institute for Clinical Excellence.

Faculty of General Dental Practitioners (UK). Selection Criteria for Dental Radiography. 2nd edn. Eds: Pendlebury ME, Horner K, Eaton KA. Royal College of Surgeons of England, London, 2004.

Scottish Intercollegiate Guidelines Network (SIGN). Management Of Unerupted and Impacted Third Molar Teeth. A National Clinical Guideline. Edinburgh: SIGN 2000.

Chapter 6
Quality Assurance in Panoramic Radiography

Aim

The aims of this chapter are to outline the principles of a quality assurance programme and to provide the practitioner with the knowledge to overcome many of the problems encountered when producing a DPR.

Outcome

At the end of this chapter, the reader should have a raised awareness of the steps required for a dedicated quality assurance programme in order to produce high-quality diagnostic images for the minimum patient radiation dose. Using this systematic approach to image production, the reader should have become familiar with the range of problems that can adversely affect panoramic image quality and have the necessary knowledge of how to rectify them.

Introduction

A high-quality DPR is produced by careful attention to the correct positioning of the patient, followed by optimum processing of the radiograph. Unfortunately, the many variables in the panoramic technique itself often conspire to lead to the production of a less than adequate final product. This can compromise or prevent diagnosis and, in the more extreme cases, negate the purpose for which the film was taken. The level of unacceptable films varies from 18.2% to 33%, with low density/low contrast films and incorrect positioning of the patient being the most common problems (Fig 6-1).

How to Overcome Problems of Poor-Quality Images

The necessity to produce a high-quality radiographic image requires a concerted effort by staff, along with the development of a dedicated Quality Assurance (QA) programme. Such a programme will ensure the production of a high quality diagnostic image with the minimum radiation dose to the patient and with limited cost to the health care provider. To achieve these ideals, a quality control programme is developed to selectively test the major

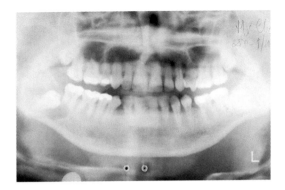

Fig 6-1 DPR with low density. The film illustrates the difficulty in diagnosis when relying on less than optimal image quality. There is a unilocular radiolucency in the right angle of the mandible overlying an unerupted third molar: a dentigerous cyst.

components of the radiographic system on a regular basis, thereby ensuring optimum performance. The major components of any radiographic system are:

- x-ray equipment
- practical radiographic technique
- image receptor (film/screen combinations, digital system)
- darkroom
- processing
- image viewing.

The routine testing of each of these components is combined with monitoring and regular auditing of the quality of the final image. There are two methods to monitor film quality:

- day-to-day surveillance
- a retrospective criterion-based clinical audit.

Most dentists continuously monitor radiographic quality during patient management. This simple method of evaluation can be improved by comparing each film to a reference or 'ideal' film. This day-to-day surveillance rapidly alerts the clinician to major departures from ideal film quality.

Some film faults are, however, more subtle, resulting in a gradual deterioration in film quality that often goes unnoticed or is unrecognised. A criterion-based clinical audit allows the practitioner to effectively identify areas of poor practice by systematically assessing each stage of image production. The audit is effective in highlighting areas of poor practice, allowing the practitioner to rapidly instigate change to improve film quality. These may include the need for equipment maintenance, an improvement in radiographic technique or the need for improved staff training. The criterion-based audit requires a standard (Table 6-1) against which the adequacy of the film can be judged. Simply looking at 'current practice' and the identification of what is wrong without measuring it against 'best practice' will obviously achieve very little. In the United Kingdom, the need to implement a suitable QA programme for dental radiography is a legal requirement. The QA programme to ensure optimum image quality should include:

- a daily film reject log
- a routine image quality assessment at six monthly intervals or immediately if film quality suddenly deteriorates

A well-designed QA programme must be inexpensive to operate, both from a monetary standpoint and with regard to the staff time involved. It should be the responsibility of a named person. The QA programme should detail the frequency with which surveys and checks of the radiographic system are to be undertaken, and this information must be kept in a written log.

Identifying the Problem – A Reject Film Analysis

Using the criteria given in Table 6-1, the practitioner can then implement a 'reject film analysis', which is in essence a subjective evaluation of film quality. Poor-quality films tend to fall into several distinct categories according to the errors present:

- poor positioning
- unsharp image
- too pale
- too dark
- low contrast.

With the exception of poor positioning, which is discussed later, each fault type, its cause(s) and the methods used for correction are detailed in Tables 6-2, 6-3, 6-4 and 6-5.

How can we Improve Panoramic Film Quality?

It is extremely important that dentists understand how their DPRs are produced so that they can 'trouble-shoot' the system. Often, film faults are unique to the individual dentist or practice and tend to recur regularly, the inference being that they are not recognised.

Table 6-1 **Quality standards for panoramic radiography** (Taken from: Radiation Protection 136: European guidelines for radiation protection in dental radiology. Luxembourg, Office for Official Publications of the European Communities, 2004.)

A: Patient preparation/instruction to patient
- Edge-to-edge incisors
- No removable metallic foreign bodies (e.g., earrings, spectacles, dentures)
- No motion artefacts
- Tongue against roof of mouth
- Minimisation of spine shadow

B: No patient positioning errors
- No antero-posterior positioning errors (equal vertical and horizontal magnification)
- No mid-sagittal plane positioning errors (symmetrical magnification)
- No occlusal plane positioning errors
- Correct positioning of spinal column

C: Correct anatomical coverage
Appropriate coverage depending upon the clinical application. Field size limitation should have been used (if available) to exclude structures irrelevant to clinical needs (e.g., limitation of field to teeth and alveolar bone for everyday dental use).

D: Good density and contrast
There should be good density and adequate contrast between the enamel and the dentine.

E: No problems with cassette or intensifying screens
- No light leaks
- Good film/screen contact
- Clean screens

F: Adequate processing and darkroom techniques
- No pressure marks on film, no emulsion scratches
- No roller marks (automatic processing only)
- No evidence of film fog
- No chemical streaks/splashes/contamination
- No evidence of inadequate fixation/washing
- Name/date/left or right marker all legible

Table 6-2 **The causes of an unsharp panoramic image**

Fault	Causes	How to remedy fault
Unsharp image	Patient movement (often occurs with younger and older patients)	Inform patient of length of exposure and the necessity to keep still.
		Assess patient prior to examination as to their degree of cooperation.
		Exclude patients with medical problems which result in uncoordinated movement (i.e., Parkinson's disease, facial dyskinesias and dystonias).
	Poor positioning	See stage 2: patient positioning
	Poor film/screen contact (cassette film)	Check hinges and catches of cassette for signs of damage.
		Check screens for signs of deterioration of screen backing support.
		Depending on the problem, order either a new cassette or replacement screens.

Table 6-3 **The causes of a pale panoramic film** Those faults relating specifically to automatic or manual processing are prefixed by letters [A] and [M], respectively.

Fault	Causes	How to remedy fault
Film too pale	***Processing fault:*** Developer solution too dilute	[M]: Discard and mix new chemistry according to manufacturer's instructions. [A]: Use solutions according to manufacturer's instructions.
	Developer too cold	[M]: Increase temperature of developer; use manufacturer's time-temperature chart. [A]: Adjust temperature control; if no change in film quality, call in specialist to repair equipment.
	Developer oxidised	[M] And [A]: Discard chemistry appropriately; replace with new chemistry.
	Developing time too short	[M]: Use manufacturer's time-temperature chart. [A]: Increase cycle time if possible; otherwise call in specialist to rectify.
	Developer contaminated by fixer	[M]: Ensure that chemicals are prepared in dedicated and labelled containers to prevent contamination [A]: Transport system contaminated. Clean immediately. Routine cleaning is recommended, follow manufacturer's instructions.
	Fixer time too long	[M]: Usually for twice the time required to develop the film.

Fault	Causes	How to remedy fault
	X-ray exposure: Incorrect x-ray exposure set	Alter exposure time.
	Failure to keep switch depressed	Keep switch depressed.
	Equipment failure: timer inaccurate, switch contact faulty, kV/mA inaccuracies	Take equipment out of service and call for engineer to service/ repair equipment.
	Film cassette positioned back to front in film carriage or upside down	Care needed in correctly positioning cassette.

Table 6-4 **The causes of a dark panoramic film** Those faults relating specifically to automatic or manual processing are prefixed by letters [A] and [M], respectively.

Fault	Causes	How to remedy fault
Film too dark	***Processing fault:*** Developer concentration too high	[M] and [A]: Dilute or change chemicals.
	Development time too long	[M]: Use time-temperature chart. [A]: Transport system has slowed down; adjust cycle time if possible. If problem does not resolve, check for wear and corrosion in equipment especially in the transport system. Call in engineer to rectify.
	Solution temperature too hot	[M]: Reduce temperature of developer; use manufacturer's time-temperature chart. [A]: Adjust temperature control; if no change in film quality, call in specialist to repair equipment.
	Contaminated solutions	Change chemistry following thorough cleaning of processor.
	Fogged film: Light leak in darkroom	Check darkroom.
	Light leak in cassette	Check hinges, catches and outer casing (especially plastic cassettes) for damage. Either effect temporary repair or take out of service and replace.

Fault	Causes	How to remedy fault
	Faulty safelighting	Check safe light visually for filter crack; check for correct bulb wattage, correct filter and correct distance above work surface. Use coin test.
	Film outdated	Discard film.
	Poor film storage: excessive temperature, excessive humidity	Discard film and designate new storage area.
	X-ray exposure: Incorrect x-ray exposure set	Alter exposure time.
	Equipment failure: timer inaccurate, switch contact faulty, kV/mA inaccuracies	Take equipment out of service and call for engineer to service/ repair equipment.

Table 6-5 **The causes of a low contrast panoramic film** Those faults relating specifically to automatic or manual processing are prefixed by letters [A] and [M], respectively.

Fault	Causes	How to remedy fault
Low contrast film	***Processing fault:*** Overdevelopment	See Table 6-4
	Underdevelopment	See Table 6-3
	Developer contaminated by fixer	Discard chemistry and start again.
	Inadequate fixation (films opaque with a milky sheen)	If processing manually it may be possible to retrieve the situation. Place film in container of fixer for 10 minutes, wash for 20 minutes and then dry. This works even if 'under-fixed' film had previously been dried. Ensure all films are fixed for the appropriate time.
		This appearance also occurs when fixer is exhausted, check date when chemistry changed.
	Fogged film	See section on film fogging in Table 6-4

The aim of the next section is to alert the practitioner to the problems associated with creating a DPR. This takes you step by step through each stage of image production. This process commences by loading the cassette in the darkroom, preparing the patient, imaging the patient, processing the film, and finally viewing the film.

At each stage, attention will be drawn to possible problems and the method of correction. In addition, the necessary quality control tests and procedures needed to ensure continuing optimum performance will be detailed along with the frequency of their implementation.

Producing a DPR

Stage 1: The Darkroom

This section relates to those practitioners who are using cassettes with screen/film combinations followed by processing in a darkroom or desktop processor.

The energy carried by the emerging x-ray beam interacts with the inorganic salts (phosphors) in the screens, causing them to fluoresce. The light emitted has, as near as possible, the same energy information as recorded by the original x-ray beam. This light exposes the photosensitive film emulsion sandwiched between the contiguous screens.

As screen film is obviously extremely sensitive to light, routine checks should be made to ensure that the darkroom is light-tight and the safe lights are 'safe'. Desktop units should be similarly checked for light tightness.

The dedicated dark room

Light may leak between the door and the doorframe or from an inadequately blacked-out window, causing exposure of the film ('light fogging'). Following processing, resultant films have low contrast and are dark, with radiopaque objects (i.e., metal restorations) appearing grey rather than clear (Fig 6-2).

When assessing the darkroom for light tightness, the inspection must be carried out in total darkness, after allowing time for the eyes to adjust. Light leaks

Fig 6-2 This DPR appears very grey and has low contrast, apart from a hand-shaped area in the lower middle part of the image. This has been produced by fogging (from poor safe lights) except in the region where the film was being held by the operator just before processing.

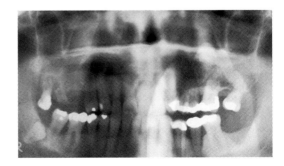

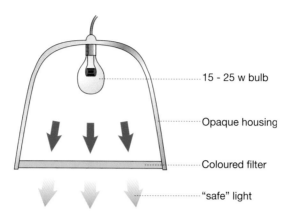

15 - 25 w bulb

Opaque housing

Coloured filter

"safe" light

Fig 6-3 A schematic to illustrate the components of a safe light.

should be clearly marked on the adjacent wall to allow their identification when the lights are subsequently turned on.

Safe lights
Processing in total darkness is not an option, so some form of lighting in the darkroom is needed. Safe lighting allows unexposed or exposed but unprocessed film to be handled without fogging. Safe lights can be positioned either 'directly' above the work surface so that 'safe light' falls on the film during the handling stage or 'indirectly' reflecting light from an adjacent ceiling or wall.

A safe light consists of a metal housing, a low-powered bulb, and a coloured filter (Fig 6-3). The part of the visible spectrum transmitted by the filter depends on the type used and should be chosen to match the colour sensitivity of the screen film in use. Different film types, whose colour sensitivity is directly related to the type of screen used, may well require different safe light conditions, and the manufacturer's recommendations should be carefully followed. Direct safe lights should be positioned 1.2m (4 feet) above the work surface and contain a low-wattage lamp (<25 W). The filter of the safe light should be periodically inspected to check for cracking or other deterioration.

The final test for safe light safety is the coin test. The test is carried out in the darkroom with the safe lights turned on. A portion of screen film, with a coin or other radiopaque object on it, is exposed to the safe light for the normal handling time of film prior to processing and then processed. If peripheral fogging highlights a clear outline of the coin, the safe lighting

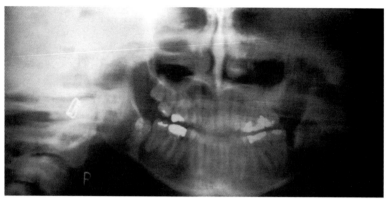

Fig 6-4 A DPR showing graduated fogging along its length The severity reflects the time spent in the loading compartment of the automatic processor before passing onto the transport system.

requires urgent rectification. The coin test can be refined using a series of coins that are sequentially uncovered at one-minute intervals to give an indication of how long the safe light is, in fact, 'safe'.

Desktop processors
Desktop processing units should be similarly checked for light tightness. These automatic systems consist of a light-tight housing with a safe light filter covering the viewing port. The safe light filter can become cracked, allowing light to leak into the processor and fog the films (Fig 6-4) as they are being loaded into the transport system. A temporary repair can be achieved by securely taping a black card over the viewing port until the replacement filter is available and can be fitted. The access sleeves are another weak point as, over time, they can become worn, allowing ingression of light. Good sense dictates that these units should never be positioned in direct sunlight or directly under bright room lights, as this can also produce film fogging.

The following checks should be carried out routinely every 12 months, immediately following any alterations to or the maintenance of safe lights, or if there have been changes to the existing light proofing to the darkroom:
• light tight: testing for the adequacy of light proofing
• safe light testing: position of safe light; correct filter used and is intact; bulb wattage correct
• a coin test.

Details of these procedures being carried out must be recorded.

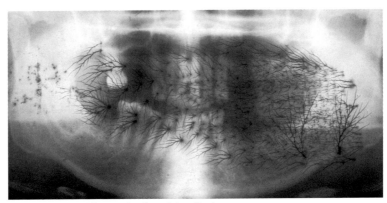

Fig 6-5 A DPR with a static electricity discharge.

Film storage and film type

Film quality is reduced by inadequate storage of film. Ideal storage conditions for screen film are in cool (<13°C), dry conditions, remote from contamination and with avoidance of pressure. The latter is achieved by storing boxed screen film in an upright position. The use of a wide-latitude film (advertised as L type) will provide maximum diagnostic information, as it records detail of both soft tissue and bony structures.

Care must also be taken when loading the film into the cassette to avoid bending. Rough or rapid handling of the film can result in a discharge of static electricity (Fig 6-5). Static presents in several ways: as a naked tree or as a smudge. The latter tends to occur more commonly when the operator is handling film wearing surgical gloves. Other causes of static are synthetic clothing and a dry atmosphere in the darkroom. Processing solutions can also contaminate films, so it is essential that all the work surfaces in the darkroom are kept meticulously clean.

Film has a definite shelf-life, as base fog increases if it is kept beyond its expiration date. The QA programme for film should include a routine three-monthly stock control to ensure out-of-date film is taken out of service Details of film stock should be recorded.

Cassettes

Cassettes incorporating intensifying screens are used routinely for extraoral radiography. The rear outer protective covering of the cassette is either a rigid aluminium lead-lined structure or is made of a flexible plastic material.

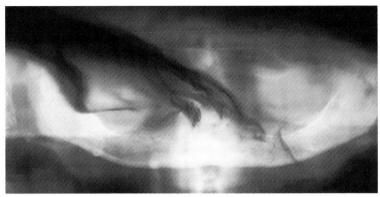

Fig 6-6 Light leaking into a split cassette as shown by black overexposed areas over the film.

The side facing the x-ray tube is made of a thin, low atomic number material to limit absorption of the emerging beam. Metal cassettes are much more robust than the plastic type, which tend to crack following prolonged use. As a consequence, light leaks into the cassette producing a localized 'fogging' of the film (Fig 6-6). These 'light leaks' can be recognised as a diffuse black area across the film mirroring the outline of the crack but extending over a slightly larger area. A temporary repair with black 'tank tape' can save the day until the new cassette arrives.

Problems with the rigid cassettes tend to be related to the clips, hinges and locking devices. If the operator fails to close the cassette correctly, or the locking mechanism fails, a blurred image is produced (Fig 6-7). Production

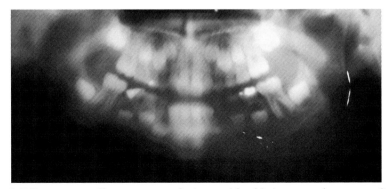

Fig 6-7 Poor screen-film contact results in considerable image unsharpness as light emission from the screens diffuses before it reaches the film.

81

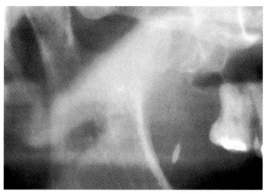

Fig 6-8 DPR with several small artefacts (small white areas) due to accumulated dust and material on the screens.

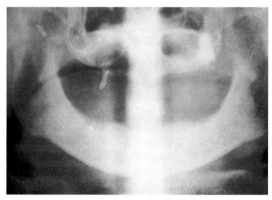

Fig 6-9 DPR with many fine artefacts over the lower part of the image due to screen cracking. Note also the larger artefact due to screen damage overlying the upper right premolar region.

of a sharp image is dependent upon the film being tightly sandwiched between the intensifying screens. If damage occurs to the locking mechanism or the supporting pressure pad of the intensifying screen, the result is poor screen–film contact. This results in considerable loss of image sharpness, caused by diffusion of light from the screens before it reaches the film. A new cassette and/or screens will rectify the problem.

The intensifying screens must be clean and undamaged to produce a sharp image. Dust particles on the screens prevent light emission and will appear as scattered white dots on the processed film (Fig 6-8). Other foreign material, such as discarded plastic film packets, paperclips (very obvious) and fragments of fabric can become trapped on the screens. Differentiation between a screen artefact and a foreign body in the patient is relatively easy, as the former has a sharp margin while the latter is diffuse.

To combat the above problems, keeping the cassette closed except when loading or unloading the film will protect the screens from acquiring foreign material and dust particles. The screens should be cleaned using the appropriate antistatic screen cleaner on a regular fortnightly basis using a soft cloth. The screens should never be soaked with the cleaning fluid, as they are hydrophilic and will subsequently crack (Fig 6-9). The cassette should be left open until the screens are dry, as premature closure will result in irreparable damage to the screens.

There appear to be no hard and fast rules as to the longevity of screens, but 10 years seems to be the upper limit for screen efficiency. If more than one cassette is in use in the practice, a unique cassette identifier (i.e., discrete markers placed at the periphery of the screen) is essential to allow a problem cassette to be identified. Similarly, 'R' and 'L' lead markers on the cassette enable correct orientation of the film.

The light sensitivity of the film should be correctly matched with the intensifying screens. Blue-sensitive film is used with calcium tungstate screens and a green-sensitive film with the faster rare-earth screens. Failure to correctly match film sensitivity to screen light emission results in the production of a low-contrast film. If you are unsure as to the type of screen phosphor in your cassette, expose the screens of an opened cassette in a darkened room and view the colour of emitted light.

The QA programme for cassettes should include a routine visual inspection of cassettes (i.e., casing, hinges, and locking mechanisms) at intervals not exceeding six months.

Stage 2: Operator Technique
Preparing the patient
Within every panoramic machine, the manufacturer builds in a defined area or layer into which the patient must be correctly positioned to achieve an undistorted image. This layer is known as the focal trough (Fig 6-10). It is elliptical in shape with three-dimensional form (i.e., height and width) replicating the shape of the 'average jaw' (i.e., Class 1). In certain types of panoramic equipment, the focal trough is narrower anteriorly than laterally, making correct positioning of the anterior teeth even more critical.

83

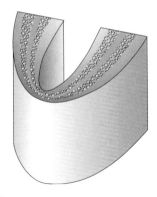

Fig 6-10 The focal trough.

As stated in Chapter 2, patients should remove bulky outdoor clothing, as it can interfere with the rotational movement of the cassette.

All radiopaque objects on the head from eye level down to the shoulder level should be removed if at all possible. Such objects include:
- dentures with radiopaque teeth and metallic components
- spectacles
- earrings
- other body piercing jewellery (e.g., nose studs, lip rings, tongue bars)
- hearing aids
- necklaces
- garments with zips/metal fasteners high on the back of the neck
- hair clips.

Earrings appear as real and ghost images (see Chapter 2), with the latter appearing as a magnified and blurred image at a higher level on the opposite side of the jaw (Fig 6-11). If the patient is unable to remove their earrings for whatever reason, turn the earring upward onto the helix/antihelix of the external ear and hold it in place with anti-allergenic tape. This ensures that the ghost image of the earring will not appear on the resultant radiograph. If radiopaque objects cannot be removed, it may be sensible to consider other types of radiography (e.g., oblique lateral views).

Positioning the patient
Modern panoramic units use a system of lights to correctly position the patient. Other additional positioning aids include combinations of some or all of the following: a chin rest, a bite block, lateral head supports, a front

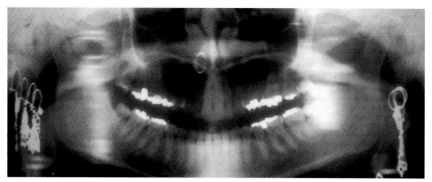

Fig 6-11 The DPR was taken without removing several earrings. Earrings appear as real and ghost images, with the latter appearing as a magnified and blurred image at a higher level on the opposite side of the jaw to the real image.

positioning guide. Many practices may have equipment without these refinements, relying instead on a bite block and/or chin rest to position the patient. Correctly positioning the patient in equipment of this type is technically more demanding.

The major factor in producing a good quality DPR is to have an understanding of how to correctly position the patient. This involves knowledge of several radiographic planes. These include the mid-sagittal plane (Fig 6-12), the inter-pupillary line (Fig 6-12), and the Frankfort plane (Fig 6-13). The latter is a plane intersecting the lower orbital border and the external auditory meatus (Fig 6-13) and should lie parallel to the floor when the patient is correctly positioned in the panoramic unit. Similarly, the interpupillary line should be parallel to the floor and the mid-sagittal plane at right angles to it. Details of how to correctly position the patient are given in Chapter 2.

There are four ways in which incorrect positioning of the patient can affect image quality. These positioning errors relate to the:
- anteroposterior position
- mid-sagittal plane
- inter-pupillary line
- occlusal plane.

Anteroposterior positioning errors
The anterior teeth become blurred if they are outside the focal trough.

85

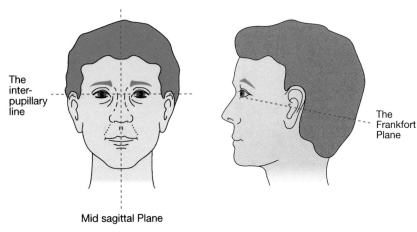

Fig 6-12 The mid-sagittal plane and the interpupillary line.

Fig 6-13 The Frankfort plane which intersects the lower orbit and the external auditory meatus.

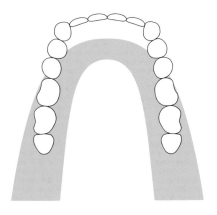

Fig 6-14 A schematic representation of positioning the patient too far forward relative to the focal trough (shaded).

When the patient's head is positioned too far forward (Fig 6-14)

The anterior teeth will appear narrow and blurred and the cervical spine will be superimposed on the ascending rami and condyles bilaterally (Fig 6-15). Additionally, the premolars will show greater horizontal overlap. There is a very obvious narrowing of the image of the jaws, as evidenced by their limited coverage on the radiograph.

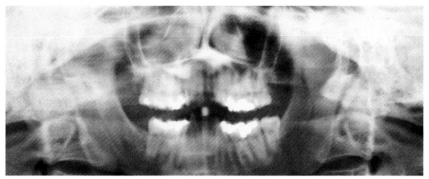

Fig 6-15 DPR with the patient positioned too far forward. The anterior teeth are extremely narrow and blurred and the cervical spine is superimposed on the ascending rami and condyles bilaterally.

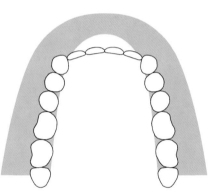

Fig 6-16 A schematic representation of positioning the patient too far back relative to the focal trough.

When the patient's head is too far back (Fig 6-16)

The anterior teeth are widened and blurred (Fig 6-17). Additionally, the TMJ region may well not be imaged in its entirety on the film. This relates especially to the condyles that may only be partially imaged on the lateral aspects of the film.

Mid-sagittal plane and interpupillary positioning errors

Mid-sagittal positioning error

The fault can involves a pure lateral rotation (Fig 6-18) of the head with the interpupillary line remaining parallel to the floor. The image shows unequal magnification of the rami and the premolars/molars, as structures nearest to the x-ray tube are magnified whilst those on the opposite side, nearest to the film, are reduced (Fig 6-19). The teeth are also often blurred and overlapped

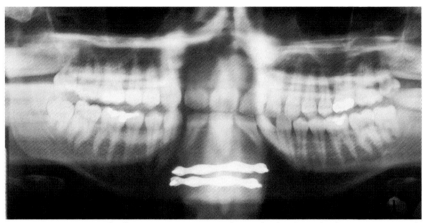

Fig 6-17 DPR with the patient positioned too far back with the anterior teeth appearing widened and blurred (note miniplates).

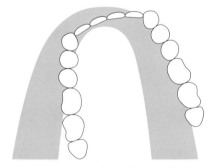

Fig 6-18 A schematic representation of a mid-sagittal positioning error. The fault involves a pure lateral rotation of the head.

because they are outside the image layer. The inferior meatus on the magnified side appears drawn out and overlies the maxillary antrum.

Mid-sagittal plane and interpupillary positioning error
The patient's head is tilted and rotated, as evidenced by the differing levels of the condyles relative to the upper edge of the film, and there is unequal magnification of the premolars/molars (Fig 6-20).

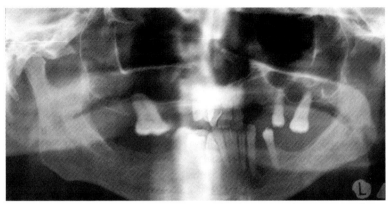

Fig 6-19 DPR with the patient's head rotated. The image shows unequal magnification of the rami and the premolar/molar teeth, as structures nearest to the x-ray tube are magnified while those on the opposite side, nearest to the film, are reduced.

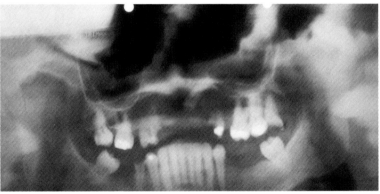

Fig 6-20 DPR with the patient's head tilted. The condyles are at different levels at the upper edge of the film and there is unequal magnification of the premolar/molar teeth. In addition, the upper aspect of the film displays light fogging due to a crack in the flexible cassette.

Occlusal plane positioning errors
Chin too far down

The patient is positioned with the Frankfort plane with a pronounced downward angulation. The DPR will show excessive curvature of the occlusal plane and the TMJ region may not be seen at the superior margin of the film (Fig 6-21). The image of the lower incisors is generally indistinct and lacks defini-

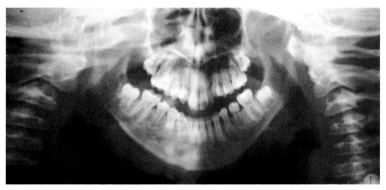

Fig 6-21 DPR with the patient's chin too far down.

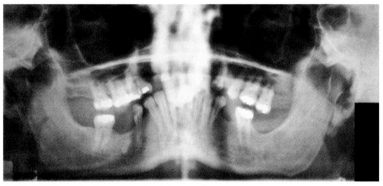

Fig 6-22 DPR with the patient's chin too far up.

tion especially in the periapical region due to this part of the tooth being positioned well outside the focal trough. The elongated ghost image of the hyoid bone is evident, being superimposed on the lower cortex of the mandible.

Chin tilted upwards
The DPR will show a flat occlusal plane and one or both condyles may not appear on the lateral aspect of the film. The maxillary anterior teeth are positioned outside the focal trough with concomitant magnification and blurring (Fig 6-22). The dense opacity of the real and ghost images of the hard palate overlie the apices of the maxillary teeth. There is often loss of the image of the condyles bilaterally from the film.

90

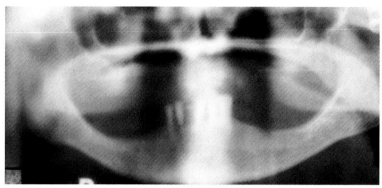

Fig 6-23 DPR with spinal column error, shown as a V-shaped radiopacity overlying the anterior maxilla and nasal region. There is also evidence of poor film–screen contact.

Other common errors
Spinal column error
The patient is allowed to slump forward in the panoramic unit rather than adopting an upright stance. The resultant film will show the dense radiopacity of the ghost image of the spine overlying and obscuring the anterior region of the jaws (Fig 6-23). This is a result of excessive absorption of radiation by the cervical spine and the associated soft tissue.

Dark radiolucent band overlying the apices of the maxillary teeth
This is a common fault caused by not instructing the patient to press their tongue to the roof of their mouth for the duration of the exposure. It is useful to prepare the patient before the exposure by asking them to swallow and hold the tongue against the palate or to 'suck in' their cheeks.

If the tongue is not positioned correctly, there is a relative overexposure of bony structures in the maxilla which obscures the apices of the maxillary teeth (Fig 6-24). If this fault occurs, 'bright lighting' the dark areas of the panoramic image using a high intensity light source shining through the film will aid diagnosis.

Dark radiolucent band overlying the premolar teeth
Not instructing the patient to close their lips around the bite block leads to the presence of bilateral air shadows overlying the maxilla and mandible. The extent of the radiolucency depends on whether the mouth is wide open (Fig

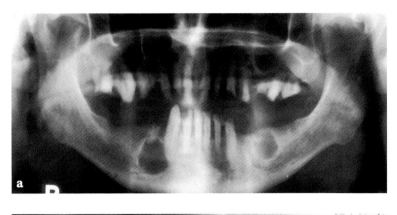

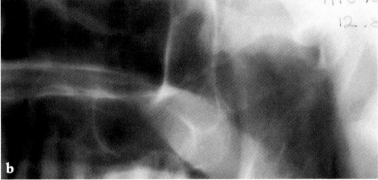

Fig 6-24 DPR with tongue not positioned adjacent to the palate. The image a) displays a gross overexposure of the maxillary region. This obscures pathology, such as the large radicular cyst in the left maxilla b) shown in this magnified portion of the DPR.

6-25) or the lips are partially closed. In the latter case, the air shadow delineated by the commisure can be mistaken for caries, typically on a lower premolar (Fig 5-5).

Distortion due to movement
Movement of the patient can be in a vertical or a horizontal direction. An up-and-down movement during the exposure is identified as a wavy undulation of the lower cortex of the mandible and a blurring of the image above this region (Fig 6-26). The patient should have been previously informed about the duration of the exposure and of the need to remain still. A sud-

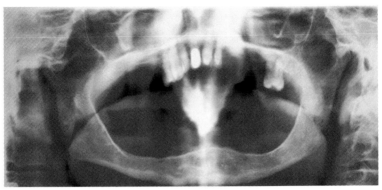

Fig 6-25 DPR taken with the patient's mouth wide open.

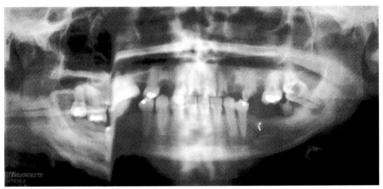

Fig 6-26 Patient made a sharp vertical movement during the rotational movement resulting in a gross irregularity of the right posterior inferior cortical border of the mandible.

den movement of the patient in a horizontal direction in the same direction as the tube can produce a double image (Fig 6-27). Panoramic radiography is not suitable for patients with medical problems (Fig 6-28) resulting in uncoordinated movements (i.e., Parkinson's disease, facial dyskinesias and dystonias).

Patient interferes with rotational movement of the cassette
Bulky clothing should be removed so that it does not interfere with the rotational movement. Certain physical attributes (i.e., a short neck and well-developed shoulders) can also interfere with the rotation of the cassette. Plac-

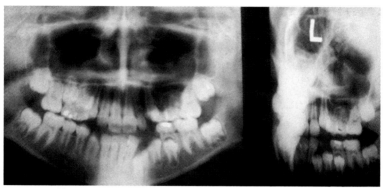

Fig 6-27 Sudden horizontal movement in the same direction of the tube resulted in a double image of the lower left canine. The lateral oblique view of the jaws taken subsequent to the DPR show a normal complement of teeth.

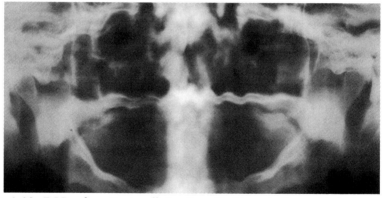

Fig 6-28 DPR of a patient suffering from Parkinson's disease displaying severe movement artefacts.

ing the cassette slightly higher and asking the patient to stretch the neck upwards can negate these problems to a degree.

Stage 3: X-Ray Equipment and the Image Receptor
X-ray equipment
The many variables of x-ray equipment (i.e., tube voltage, tube current, beam filtration, beam dimension, timer operation and radiographic output) should be examined to establish a baseline for the QA programme. X-ray equipment must be in good mechanical and electrical order and must

undergo regular maintenance and testing to ensure optimum performance. Routine checks (preferrably daily) should be carried out to assess the panoramic unit for signs of damage, in particular to the tube head. Failure of the rotational movement and/or the safety cut-out switches should be dealt with immediately by isolating the equipment and taking it out of service until the fault(s) have been rectified.

The standards set and the frequency of the tests (i.e., electrical, mechanical, output and radiation protection) will vary from country to country and are outside the remit of this book. In the United Kingdom, routine tests should be performed on x-ray equipment at least every three years. If image quality is routinely poor or the QA programme indicates significant equipment problems, then equipment testing must be undertaken immediately. Details of routine testing should be retained, as should the maintenance record of the x-ray equipment.

The image receptor
The two image receptors used in panoramic radiography are:
- cassettes containing intensifying screens for conventional imaging
- CCD and PSP receptors for digital imaging (and the TV monitors used for image display).

Cassettes containing intensifying screens
Cassettes should be routinely checked for:
- damage to the outer casing allowing light to ingress (see Stage 1: The darkroom)
- failure of compression/support pads of screens or locking mechanism leading to poor screen–film contact (see Stage 1: the darkroom)

CCD and PSP receptors
Digital panoramic equipment is becoming more commonplace in general dental practice. The advantages of such systems include immediate image display on the computer monitor and the fact that no processing chemicals or equipment are necessary. In digital systems, an assessment of spatial resolution, grey-scale resolution and signal-to-noise ratio is needed to measure image quality in an objective manner.

CCD receptors are essentially an integral part of the x-ray equipment and need no specific routine checks other than those carried out at routine servicing by a qualified engineer. PSP imaging plates superficially appear similar to the cassettes used for conventional film radiography. They will, however, not suffer the problems described above for cassettes. The principal problems that might be anticipated are scratches and related damage to the plate surface during handling.

The minimum resolution of the monitor should be 1024 x 768 pixels. The screen size of the monitor should be at least 17 inches for a conventional monitor and 15 inches for a flat-panel monitor. The grey level resolution should be set to at least 'High Colour' (16 bit), in order to display small contrasts. Brightness and contrast should be checked and adjusted to allow all grey values between black and white to be displayed correctly. Low ambient light levels are essential to fully evaluate the TV monitor image. A method of backup for image data should be available and used.

Stage 4: Film Processing
Having produced the ideal latent image, poor processing can result in the loss of important diagnostic information in the final image. QA standards for processing are clearly stated by the manufacturers of processing solutions and equipment. This information covers:
- processing conditions (time and temperatures)
- changing frequency for processing solutions
- cleaning instructions for automatic processors.

The QA programme should ensure that these standards are adhered to by recording:
- the frequency of chemical changes
- the frequency for cleaning the automatic processor.

Manual processing
When preparing chemistry, the manufacturer's dilution factors should be carefully observed. The availability of two labelled funnels and containers ensure that developer and fixer are not contaminated during their preparation. Tanks should have lids to limit evaporation and contamination of the chemistry and, in the case of the developer tank, to limit oxidation. Solution levels should be checked regularly and topped up as and when necessary.

Solutions should be given time to reach their working temperature and stirred thoroughly prior to use to ensure an even temperature throughout the tank. An accurate thermometer and a timer are essential equipment in the darkroom in order to faithfully adhere to the manufacturer's stated time/temperature relationship for optimum processing. During processing, films should be agitated periodically to disperse any attached air bubbles and to allow fresh chemistry to contact the emulsion. The important points of manual processing are detailed in Table 6-6.

The QC programme for manual processing should include detailed records of:
- the frequency of changing processing solutions
- the results of a twice-weekly audit of processing techniques (i.e., a record of developer temperature, developer time and fixer time).

Automatic processing
Although automatic processors can standardise many of the variables involved in manual processing, they are not a panacea. The long-term reliability of automatic processors is dependent upon both routine maintenance of the unit and regular cleaning. The chemical and wash tanks must be

Table 6-6 **Requirements for manual processing**

- Developer must be prepared according to dilution factors specified by manufacturer.

- Development is time/temperature specific: follow manufacturer's instructions. (These should also be detailed in the darkroom.)

- Developer has a limited shelf life and rapidly becomes oxidised. Use step wedge test to assess activity of developer.

- Solutions should be given time to reach their working temperature and stirred prior to use to ensure an even temperature throughout the tank.

- During processing, films should be agitated to disperse any attached air bubbles and to allow fresh chemistry to contact the emulsion.

- Wash films briefly following development to reduce over-carry of alkaline developer into acid fixer.

- Films must remain in fixer for twice the development time.

- Final wash for 20 minutes in running water.

- Films must be completely dry before storage.

drained and cleaned, preferably each time the chemistry is changed. The warm temperatures in the wash tank encourage algae growth that may, if left undisturbed, lead to blockage of the drainage system.

It is important to clean the film transport system (as directed by the manufacturer), as the buildup of chemical residues on the tracking can lead to chemical contamination of films. The routine use of proprietary film cleaners at the start of each day will help to remove contaminants.

The QC programme for automatic processing should include a detailed record of:
• the frequency of the changing of processing solutions
• the frequency of routine cleaning of the automatic processor
• routine servicing of the automatic processor.

Monitoring of film processing
It is essential to monitor processing to ensure optimum film quality. There are several proprietary test objects on the market that employ a step wedge with which to monitor film quality. The test object is routinely radiographed, using identical exposure parameters and focus-to-object distance. The baseline reference film is obtained following the preparation of new chemistry and subsequent processing using optimum processing conditions. Subsequently, monitoring radiographs should be produced daily (or at least twice weekly) and compared to the baseline reference film. Any alteration in step wedge density necessitates immediate action. This change can be the result of either deterioration in processing chemistry or an x-ray equipment fault. The former is more common than the latter, but processing errors must be excluded before an equipment fault is considered.

The QA programme for monitoring processing should include:
• a record of chemical stock
• details of radiographic monitoring giving details of results and action taken.

Stage 5: Viewing the Radiograph
Ideal viewing conditions are essential in order to obtain maximum diagnostic yield from the radiograph. This requires the use of a dental light box and a method of magnifying the image by a factor of two. Films should be viewed away from strong light sources.

The QC programme for monitoring light boxes should be carried out at intervals not exceeding six months and should include an assessment of:
- the glass of the light box for damage
- a routine schedule for cleaning the viewing surface of the light box
- bulb(s): checked for constant light intensity.

Reporting of radiographs
Within the UK, it is a legal requirement that every radiograph must be evaluated and an appropriate report on the radiological findings made as part of the clinical records. This reporting of films is also amenable to audit.

Conclusions

The adoption of and adherence to a quality assurance programme should ensure the routine production of high quality images.

Further Reading

Guidance Notes for Dental Practitioners on the Safe Use of X-Ray Equipment. National Radiological Protection Board. London, Department of Health, 2001.

Langland, OE, Langlais, RP, McDavid, WD and DelBalso, AM. Panoramic Radiology. 2nd Edn. Philadelphia: Lea & Febiger, 1989.

Langland OL, Langlais RP and Preece JW. Principles of Dental Imaging. 2nd Edn. Baltimore: Lippincott Williams & Wilkins, 2002.

White SC and Pharoah MJ. Oral Radiology 5th Edn. St. Louis: Mosby 2004.

Chapter 7
Radiographic Interpretation of Disease

Aim

The aims of this chapter are to:
- outline the principles of interpretation of DPRs
- describe some of the disorders that the general dental practitioner may encounter on DPRs in clinical practice. However, it is not the intention of this chapter to provide a comprehensive account of abnormalities of the jaws.

Outcome

After studying this chapter, the reader should have a basic understanding and knowledge of the radiographic features of the more common conditions that affect the teeth and jaws.

Introduction

Radiographic interpretation is the process in which information is gleaned from radiographs. Radiographs are an adjunct to the clinical examination and form part of the diagnostic process. They provide information about disease though its radiographic features. In addition, they are helpful in treatment planning and patient management.

In order to interpret radiographs it is important to have an understanding of the science of image formation. A brief outline follows, but for a fuller account the reader is referred to Chapter 1 of 'Interpreting Dental Radiographs' by Horner et al. (2002), and other more detailed texts.

Image Formation

Images are formed on radiographs because of differential absorption of x-ray photons as they pass through the tissues. X-ray absorption is proportional to the cube of the atomic number (Z^3) of the absorber and to its density, but inversely proportional to the cube of the photon energy of the x-ray beam ($1/E^3$). High atomic number or dense substances such as gold or enamel are more radiopaque than less dense or lower atomic number materials such as dentine, the soft tissues and, in particular, air, which show varying degrees of radiolucency. So the radiographic image is made up of a range of shadows of different shades of grey, depending on the physical make-up of the tissues and the exposure factors used.

The image of a DPR consists of a zone of sharpness that corresponds to the shape of the jaws. This curved focal trough is narrower anteriorly than posteriorly. Only those objects in the centre of this layer are accurately depicted whilst objects at the margins of the focal are blurred and distorted (see Chapter 6).

When examining a DPR, it is important to bear in mind that the image has less resolution than of intraoral radiographs. This is because:
- the intraoral radiographic image is formed directly on the film emulsion, whereas in dental panoramic radiography the image is formed mainly by light emitted from the intensifying screens. This light diffuses in all directions from the screens before reaching the film, resulting in a degree of blurring.
- the panoramic process involves movement which inherently produces some unsharpness, whereas there is no movement of tube or film in intraoral radiography.

Principles of Radiographic Interpretation

It is all too easy in a busy surgery to hold a radiograph up to a bright room light or a window and give the radiograph a cursory glance. Whilst this approach may reveal gross radiographic features, more subtle diagnostic information can be missed.

So How Should One Examine a DPR?

It is important to study any radiograph both systematically and thoroughly. A suggested scheme is listed below.

Use appropriate viewing conditions
A light box, which:
- has even illumination of optimal brightness (remember that a fluorscent tube gradually looses brightness and so requires periodic replacement)
- is well maintained, and clean
- is large enough to accommodate the whole film
- has a high intensity light source to examine dark areas of the film

Exclude or mask off light peripheral to the radiograph to reduce glare. This permits the pupils to dilate allowing the eyes to gather more information.

Where possible view radiographs in subdued, ambient lighting in a quiet distraction free environment.

Use magnification. Although this is particularly pertinent to examining intra-oral radiographs, it is also helpful when viewing problem areas on DPRs.

Examining radiographs in this way is less tiring on the eyes, improves radiographic contrast and maximises radiographic detail.

Be familiar with the normal panoramic image
It is essential to be able to recognise normal anatomical structures and variations of normal features in order to identify an abnormality. This includes both the hard and soft tissues, ghost shadows and image artefacts that occur with DPRs (Chapter 3).

Assess image quality (see Chapter 6)
Poor image quality results in loss of diagnostic information. This can arise from inappropriate film processing or exposure factors producing radiographs that are excessively pale or dark, whereas inaccurate radiographic technique results in image distortion.

Examine the radiograph systematically
- Use continuous eye movements rather than staring at one point.
- Follow or trace all anatomical outlines checking for discontinuity, displacement or destruction. This usually requires several 'trips' around the film.
- Check for lack of symmetry by comparing left and right sides and if present decide whether it is significant.

Familiarise yourself with disorders of the jaws
It is important to have an understanding and knowledge of the diseases that affect the jaws, their histogenesis and behaviour. For example, radicular cysts show unicystic growth, expand equally in all directions and appear round, whilst keratocysts are elongated because they enlarge along the cancellous bone due to difficulty in resorbing and expanding the cortical plates. Odontogenic disorders arise in or are centred on the alveolar parts of the jaws, so an abnormality confined to the basal bone is probably not of odontogenic origin.

Relate what you see to the clinical findings
Age, gender, race, the clinical history, the clinical examination and the results of special tests provide useful information for radiographic diagnostic process.

Use previous radiographs
These provide information on the presence or absence of pre-existing disease and on the progression of existing disease.

When examining a DPR, remember the limitations inherent in the panoramic image. It is a very useful view for many conditions, but don't forget that additional views may be needed to obtain a fuller picture. For example, a view at right angles (e.g. lower true occlusal view) to show jaw expansion, or parallax views to assist with location of unerupted teeth or foreign bodies may be needed.

This chapter now briefly describes some of the conditions that can appear on DPRs, under the following headings:
• Disorders of the teeth
• Disorders affecting the jaws
• Disorders in the soft tissues
• Disorders of the maxillary antrum
• Disorders of the temporomandibular joint.

Disorders of the Teeth

Hypodontia
This is a developmental condition in which one or more teeth fail to form. It is more prevalent in the permanent dentition (<7% excluding wisdom teeth) than the primary dentition (<1%). It particularly affects third molars, lower second premolars and maxillary lateral incisors. Its severity varies from absence of one tooth (common) to complete failure of development of the dentition or anodontia (rare).

Absence of a permanent successor often leads to prolonged retention of the primary predecessor. This can result in ankylosis of the primary molars, which may then submerge due to bone remodelling. Fig 7-1 shows a patient with hypodontia.

Certain syndromes are associated with hypodontia, some of which are outlined in Table 7-1.

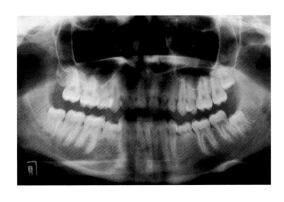

Fig 7-1 Hypodontia. The upper lateral incisors, upper and lower second premolar, and the upper right wisdom tooth are absent. There is retention of the upper primary canines and lateral incisor, and the lower primary second molars.

Table 7-1 **Syndromes associated with hypodontia**

Disorder	Associated features
Ectodermal dysplasia	Numerous missing teeth, conically shaped teeth, hypotrichosis, hypohidrosis, saddle-shaped nose
Down syndrome (Trisomy 21)	Maxillary hypoplasia, delayed cognitive skills, hearing and vision defects, cardiac abnormalities.

Hyperdontia

The condition in which there are teeth additional to the normal series is referred to as hyperdontia, or supernumerary teeth. It affects approximately 1% of the population and occurs mainly in the permanent dentition, particularly in the upper central incisor, and the molar and premolar regions of the jaws.

The types of supernumerary teeth are summarised in Table 7-2. Supernumerary teeth in the maxillary midline region may be poorly displayed on DPRs if unfavourably positioned in relation to the image layer. However, supernumeraries in the posterior regions are usually well shown on DPRs (Figs 7-2 and 7-3).

Whilst supernumerary teeth may be an isolated anomaly, they are also found in certain systemic disorders, e.g. Gardner's syndrome and cleidocranial dys-

Table 7-2 **Types of supernumerary teeth**

Type	Location	Appearance	Features
Mesiodens	Either side of the midline of the maxilla	Small and conically shaped	Occurs singly or paired. Can erupt, invert, or prevent eruption of the permanent incisor. Develops chronologically between that of the primary and permanent central incisors.
Tuberculate	Either side of the midline of the maxilla, usually palatally located	Small, cusped tooth	Can occur singly or paired. Develops chronologically shortly after the permanent central incisors, and usually prevents their eruption.
Supplemental premolars	Mainly premolar or molar regions	Resembles normal premolars or molars	Develops shortly after the adjacent permanent teeth, often remain unerupted.
Paramolars	Adjacent to the molar teeth	Small and rudimentary	Situated buccal or lingual to a maxillary molar
Disto-molars	Distal to the wisdom teeth	Often small and conical	Occasionally erupt

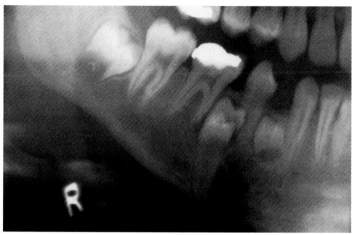

Fig 7-2 Two supplemental supernumeraries at an early stage of development and a displaced, unerupted lower right second premolar.

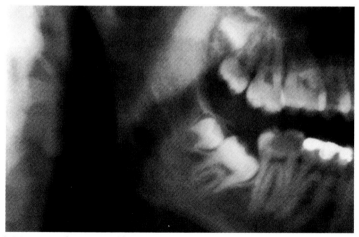

Fig 7-3 Unerupted upper and lower distomolar with incomplete root development. The lower right third molar is impacted and the second molar is grossly decayed.

plasia (Fig 7-4). Cleidocranial dysplasia is associated with multiple supernumerary and unerupted teeth (Fig 7-4).

Impacted Third Molars
Lower wisdom teeth often fail to fully erupt because of insufficient room to

Table 7-3 **Radiographs used to assess wisdom teeth**

Technique	Advantages	Disadvantages
DPR	Shows all four wisdom teeth.	Relative lack of image definition.
	Shows full depth of mandible.	Long exposure time-patient must keep still.
	Good patient compliance.	Dose may be larger than periapical views
Oblique lateral mandible	Alternative to DPR.	Relative lack of image definition.
	Shows upper and lower wisdom teeth on one side.	Short exposure time.
	Technique simple with good patient compliance.	Some image distortion.
Periapical radiographs	Good image definition.	Poor patient acceptance due to lack of depth and sensitivity of lingual sulcus.
	Useful for examining single wisdom tooth.	
	Vertical parallax views can be used to help identify position on the IDC.	Unsuitable for patients with a tendency to gag or limited mouth opening.
		Not suitable for deeply placed wisdom teeth.
	Widely available.	

accommodate them into the dental arch. Impacted, partially erupted wisdom teeth are prone to develop caries and/or pericoronitis. Although the DPR is usually perceived as the most appropriate view to image impacted wisdom teeth, there are alternatives views. (Table 7-3).

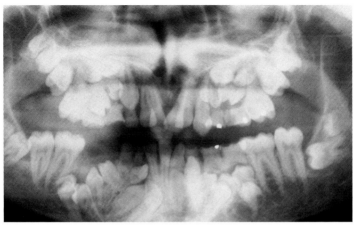

Fig 7-4 Cleidocranial dysplasia, showing numerous unerupted permanent and supernumerary teeth. Very few of the permanent teeth have erupted.

The radiographic assessment of impacted wisdom teeth has been described in Chapter 8 of 'Interpreting Dental Radiographs' by Horner et al. 2002, to which the reader is referred. For ease of reference, a scheme is outlined below that contains the key features for assessing an impacted lower wisdom tooth.

Nature of impaction
- type of impaction; soft tissue, tooth, bone, or a combination of these.
- angulation of impaction, relative to that of the vertical axis of the lower second molar. The types are: horizontal, mesio-angular, vertical, disto-angular, transverse (rare). Whilst horizontal impactions may look difficult, disto-angularly impacted wisdom teeth often prove troublesome to remove, due to the close approximation of the roots of the wisdom tooth to the second molar roots and the lack of access and space to deliver the tooth.

Status of crown
Assess whether sound, carious and/or bulbous. Decay is common in those teeth susceptible to food stagnation, notably partly erupted, mesio-angular or horizontally impacted wisdom teeth.

Root morphology (Fig 7-5)
- stage of root development
- number of roots

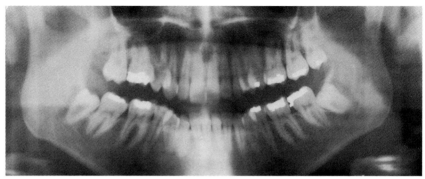

Fig 7-5 Both lower wisdom teeth in this patient are mesio-angularly impacted, the lower right having a conical root, the apices lying close to the inferior alveolar canal.

- curvature
- size
- bulbosity
- proximity to the inferior alveolar canal.

Wisdom teeth with roots that are short and conical are easier to remove than those with multiple, long and curved roots.

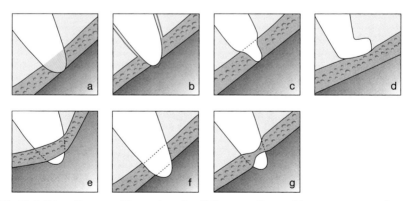

Fig 7-6 Line diagrams illustrating the different radiographic appearances of roots grooved by the inferior alveolar canal. a) change of density (radiolucency) of the root; b) loss of lamina dura around the root where it is crossed by the canal; c) constriction or narrowing of the root; d) curvature or hooking of the root where it abuts up against the roof of the canal; e) change in direction of the canal as it crosses the root; f) loss of one or both of the cortical outlines (tramlines) of the canal; g) constriction or narrowing of the canal.

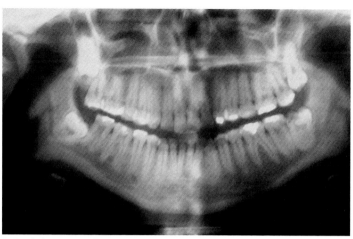

Fig 7-7 Both lower wisdom teeth roots are grooved by the inferior alveolar canal. Note the deviation of the canal on the right side and the radiolucent band at the root apex of the lower left wisdom tooth where it is crossed by the canal. The lower left wisdom tooth is carious.

Association with the inferior alveolar (dental) canal
It is essential to determine the proximity of the root to the inferior alveolar canal. An association is present if there is change to the root where it is crossed by the canal, or change to the canal where it crosses the root. These changes are depicted diagrammatically in Fig 7-6. An example of a close relationship of tooth and canal is shown in Fig 7-7.

Other features to assess
- Depth of tooth in bone/bone level; the amount of bone covering the crown.
- Density of the investing bone, the size of the marrow spaces and the number of bony trabeculae.
- Size of follicular space; normally 1 to 2 mm, but often enlarges following recurrent pericoronitis. If wider than 5 mm, indicates pathological change, such as dentigerous cyst formation.
- Condition of the remaining dentition, in particular presence of dental caries and periodontal bone loss.

Maxillary Canines
After the third molar, the maxillary canine is the second commonest tooth to fail to erupt, with up to 2% of the population being affected. During its eruption it is guided into position by the distal aspect of the root of the maxillary lateral incisor. By the age of 10 years, the crown of the unerupted canine

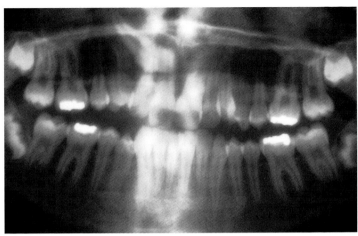

Fig 7-8 A DPR showing how position of ectopic teeth will influence their image on the DPR. In this case the right canine is widened (palatal position) and the left canine narrowed (buccal position).

is usually palpable as a smooth, domed expansion of the buccal alveolus. If the canine is not palpable by this time, it is probable that its eruption is abnormal and so requires further investigation to confirm its presence, to assess the likelihood of its eruption and whether treatment is required to assist its eruption. An intra-oral view (or parallax views) may be all that is required, but a DPR is indicated when it necessary to assess other unerupted teeth, as for example with orthodontic treatment planning.

Whilst a DPR will image unerupted canines, it may be of limited value for those teeth that are not completely located within the focal trough.

Radiographic assessment should include:
<u>Position:</u>
An unerupted maxillary canine may be placed, palatally, buccally or lie in the arch.

On a DPR, the width (mesio-distal dimension) may be used to determine the position of a canine in the arch. Assuming there is no radiographic distortion, if the canine appears wider than normal (compare with the contralateral erupted canine) it suggests that it lies palatally. This is because objects on the medial aspect of the focal trough appear magnified (and also less sharp). The converse is also true, i.e., a buccally displaced tooth will appear narrower than normal (Fig 7-8).

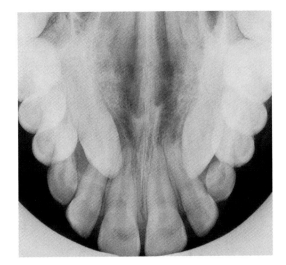

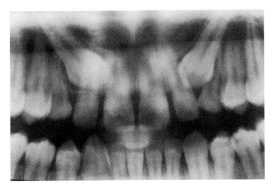

Fig 7-9 a) Upper anterior occlusal view showing two unerupted maxillary canines and b) DPR of the same patient. The tube angle for the occlusal film is 60-65° downwards, but approximately 8° upwards for the DPR. Note that the crowns of both canines are located higher up the lateral incisor root (closer to the apex) on the occlusal film 7.9.a, when compared with the DPR. Thus, they are seen to move in the same direction (downwards) as the tube angulation changes from the occlusal to the DPR, so confirming its palatal displacement.

Although the width of a maxillary canine image on a DPR is a useful guide to its location, confirmation may still be required. This can be achieved by taking an upper occlusal radiograph of the canine, which is viewed by placing it above the panoramic film and parallax applied in a vertical direction (Fig 7-9, a and b). In parallax, two views are taken of the same area but with a different tube angulation. If the object (canine crown) moves in the same direction as that taken by the tube shift relative to a fixed object (lateral incisor root) it lies palatally, whilst if it moves in the opposite direction to that taken by the tube, it will lie on the buccal side.

Note the degree of angulation of the canine relative to the adjacent teeth and the amount of space between the adjacent teeth.

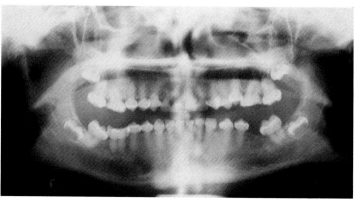

Fig 7-10 Dentinogenesis imperfecta. Note the bulbous crowns and short stumpy roots.

Crown
- Caries
- Resorption
- Examine the size of the surrounding follicular space. If its width exceeds 5 mm, is likely to be due to pathological change, such as a dentigerous cyst.

Root
- Stage of root development, a tooth with an open apex will still have eruptive potential.
- Root length and curvature.

Bone
- Assess the depth of the canine from the alveolar crest level. The DPR or, in particular, a paralleling technique periapical, will give a truer indication of depth than an upper oblique occlusal or bisected angle periapical view which exaggerate the depth of a palatally displaced canine.
- Note the bone density by checking the size of the marrow spaces. The more numerous and closer the trabeculae are packed, the more dense the bone and the less yielding it will be, should the tooth require removal.

Adjacent teeth
- Look for root resorption of the lateral incisor root. This is most likely to occur during the eruptive period of the canine. After closure of the canine root apex, resorption becomes much less likely.
- Note root length of the deciduous canine, if present
- Assess the presence of caries and periodontal status

Buried maxillary canines may not be detected until well into adulthood. Provided that they are not associated with disease, such teeth are often best left undisturbed.

Dentinogenesis Imperfecta
This is a genetically determined condition that affects dentine formation in the primary and permanent dentition.

Clinical features
The abnormal dentine gives the teeth an opalescent bluish/brown colour. The enamel tends to chip off and the crowns show marked attrition. Occasionally, the condition is associated with osteogenesis imperfecta, in which the bones are prone to fracture. There are several subdivisions of dentinogenesis imperfecta, depending on its variable presentation and associated conditions.

Radiographic features
The typical radiographic appearance is shown in Fig 7-10. The teeth have bulbous crowns and short roots. There is obliteration of the pulp chambers by abnormal dentine formation.

Periodontal Disease
It is not the remit of this book to describe periodontal disease. For an account on periodontal disease see 'Quintessentials 1' by Chapple and Gilbert.

As discussed in Chapter 5, in most cases periodontal bone loss is better assessed with intraoral radiographs (bitewing and/or periapicals) than a DPR. However, current guidelines from the Faculty of General Dental Practitioners (UK) suggest that DPRs may be used where there are other concurrent dental problems (e.g. partially erupted third molars requiring treatment) or where there is a dose advantage over multiple intraoral films (and where only a gross assessment is considered necessary). An example of a patient with rapidly progressive periodontitis is shown in Fig 7-11.

Disorders Affecting the Jaws

The radiological examination of a lesion in the jaws should be undertaken methodically. A suggested scheme is as follows:
- Identify its radiodensity; it may be:
    - Radiolucent, e.g. radicular cyst
    - Radiopaque, e.g. sclerosing osteitis
    - Mixed density e.g. cemento-ossifying fibroma

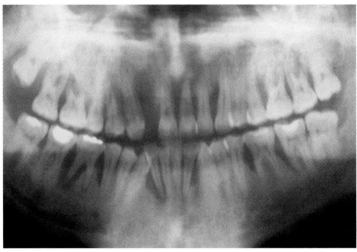

Fig 7-11 Rapidly progressive adult periodontitis with several deep infra-bony pockets. The radiograph shows the corresponding vertical bone defects.

- Note the 'Four S's':
  - Site – anatomical location, e.g. periapical region
  - Size – measured in mms or its anatomical extent
  - Shape – e.g. round, ovoid, irregular, loculated
  - Surface (outline) – e.g. well defined, ill defined, lobulated

If well defined, check whether there is a visible cortical margin (a thin radiopaque edge); this feature is associated with benign or slow-growing lesions. Ill-defined margins are associated with malignant and infected lesions. Alternatively some conditions (e.g. myeloma) appear punched out and non-corticated.

- Note the effect on adjacent structures, e.g. tooth displacement, jaw expansion, root resorption.

Well Defined Radiolucencies of the Jaws

Radicular Cyst

This is the most common of the odontogenic cysts. It is an inflammatory lesion, which arises from chronic irritation of the periapical tissues from endotoxins produced by bacteria within a non-vital root canal. Initially a granuloma forms which, if left untreated, may undergo cystic change. Many

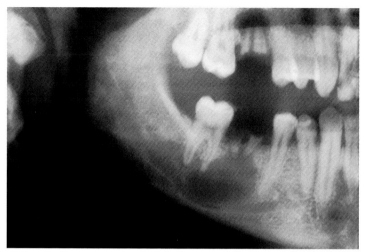

Fig 7-12 A radicular cyst associated with the roots of the lower right first molar. There is displacement of the inferior alveolar canal. There is a radiolucency at the apices of the upper right first molar which is either an apical granuloma or radicular cyst.

radicular cysts are small and best imaged on intraoral radiographs, but when large a DPR may be required to show the entire lesion.

Clinical features
Small radicular cysts are asymptomatic unless infected. Larger lesions may give rise to jaw expansion and become noticed by the patient. The causative tooth is non-vital and so may appear grossly decayed, heavily restored or has suffered previous trauma.

Radiological features
A radicular cyst (Fig 7-12) typically appears as a circular or ovoid, radiolucency, which is well defined with a cortical margin. It develops at a tooth apex where there is loss of the lamina dura, the remainder of the lamina dura being continuous with the outline of the cyst. Large radicular cysts may cause tooth displacement and jaw expansion. Of course, periapical radiolucencies are extremely common but only a minority are cystic. Furthermore it is not possible to differentiate between a radicular cyst, granuloma or chronic periapical abscess when the radiolucency is less than 15–20 mm in diameter. Lesions considered in differential diagnosis of radicular cyst are described in Table 7-4.

Table 7-4 **Differential diagnosis of a periapical radiolucency**

Disorder	Important characteristics	Radiographic features
Periapical granuloma	Associated with a non-vital tooth. Painless unless infected. Account for 50–70% of apical inflammatory radiolucencies	Ovoid in shape. Well to moderately well defined. Does not exceed 20 mm in diameter. Loss of apical lamina dura.
Chronic apical abscess	As for granuloma, but less common, incidence 10–20% of apical radiolucencies associated with non-vital teeth	As for periapical granuloma.
Radicular cyst	As for granuloma, but less common (20 – 40%). Produces jaw expansion when large.	Round in shape. Well defined, often corticated. Can exceed 20 mm in diameter. Can cause tooth displacement. Loss of apical lamina dura.
Scar tissue	Asymptomatic, history of apical surgery,	Densely radiolucent due to defect in cortical bone, may have irregular shape, rarely exceeds 10 mm in diameter.
Periapical cemento-osseous dysplasia	Occurs mainly in women, especially of Afro-Caribbean origin. Painless, multiple lesions and the associated teeth are usually vital.	Depends on stage of development. Initial stage is radiolucent. Becomes increasingly radiopaque as it matures with mineral deposited centrally.

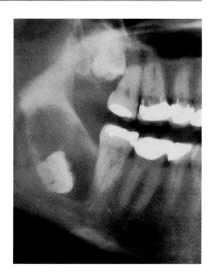

Fig 7-13 Dentigerous cyst. A well defined radiolucency enveloping the crown of an unerupted and displaced lower right wisdom tooth.

Dentigerous Cyst

The dentigerous cyst (follicular cyst) results from cystic transformation of the reduced internal and external enamel epithelium, which make up part of the tooth follicle. Enlargement of the follicular space beyond 5mm is usually regarded as the threshold indicating that pathological change has occurred. In a dentigerous cyst, the crown lies wholly or partly within the cyst lumen.

Clinical features

A dentigerous cyst is usually asymptomatic but it will become painful if it becomes infected. Alternatively, it may enlarge sufficiently to cause jaw expansion. There will be a missing tooth from the arch.

Radiological features

Typically the cyst appears as a well-defined unilocular, circular or oval, radiolucency with a corticated margin, encircling the crown of an unerupted tooth (Fig 7-13). The cyst can reach a considerable size and cause thinning and expansion of the cortical bone. Although any unerupted tooth may be affected by dentigerous cyst formation, it most frequently involves lower third molars and maxillary canines. Any well defined, radiolucent lesion that encroaches upon the crown of an unerupted tooth may resemble a dentigerous cyst, including odontogenic keratocyst, ameloblastoma or ameloblastic fibroma. However, unlike a dentigerous cyst, the crown lies outside the lesion, but this may not be apparent from the radiograph.

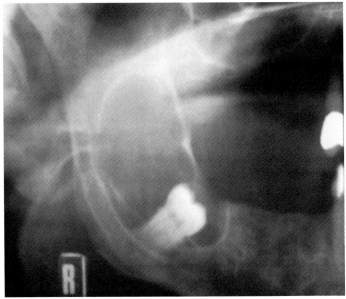

Fig 7-14 Odontogenic keratocyst in the lower right wisdom tooth region. Note the elongated shape and scalloped margin.

Odontogenic Keratocyst
This is a developmental cyst that arises from remnants of the dental lamina.

Clinical features
It is usually asymptomatic, unless infected. It has a bimodal presentation, occurring most often during the second/third or fifth/sixth decades of life. In most cases, the cyst does not produce significant bony expansion.

Radiological features
An odontogenic keratocyst appears as a radiolucency, found most often in the posterior body of the mandible, although some occur anteriorly, and the maxilla can also be affected. It has difficulty in resorbing the cortical bone and so grows along the cancellous bone to appear elongated in shape. Its margins are well defined, often corticated and scalloped, as shown in Fig 7-14. Some odontogenic keratocysts contain thin bony septa resulting in a multilocular appearance. Occasionally it develops between the roots of adjacent teeth to resemble a lateral periodontal cyst. Keratocysts have a high recurrence rate, thus long-term follow-up is essential.

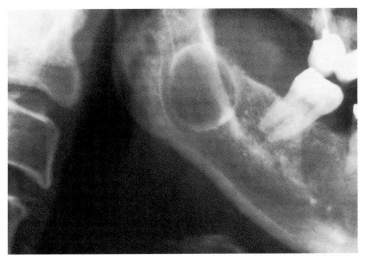

Fig 7-15 Residual cyst in the lower right wisdom tooth region.

Multiple keratocysts are a feature of Gorlin-Goltz syndrome (naevoid basal cell carcinoma syndrome). This is an uncommon but important condition, which is inherited as an autosomal dominant trait. The syndrome consists of a number of abnormalities, including frontal bossing, palmar pits, multiple naevoid basal cell carcinomas of the skin, calcification of the cerebral falx and skeletal malformations, e.g. bifid ribs.

Residual cyst
A radicular cyst that persists following the extraction of the causative tooth is referred to as a residual cyst.

Clinical features
It mainly affects adults, the incidence increasing with age. It is asymptomatic unless it becomes infected.

Radiological features
Residual cysts occur in an edentulous part of the jaws. Most are slow growing, or show no growth, although a few can achieve considerable size, as shown in Fig 7-15. Typically, a residual cyst appears as a round, well-defined radiolucency with a cortical margin. Long-standing residual cysts may show dystrophic mineralisation, which appear as radiopaque foci.

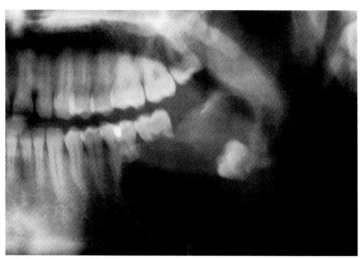

Fig 7-16 Cystic ameloblastoma. Note the marked root resorption of the lower left first and second molars.

Ameloblastoma
The ameloblastoma is a tumour of odontogenic epithelium that accounts for about 11% of odontogenic tumours. Although benign, it is locally aggressive and requires wide excision. There is a rare but malignant form.

Clinical features
The ameloblastoma is a slow-growing tumour usually discovered during the fourth or fifth decades of life. When small it is asymptomatic but when large can produce discomfort, swelling and tooth mobility. Most (80%) ameloblastomas occur in the posterior body of the mandible. The unicystic ameloblastoma is a variant of the ameloblastoma that arises in the wall of a pre-existing cyst. It usually occurs in the second or third decades of life.

Radiographic features
The ameloblastoma has a variable appearance but typically appears as a multilocular, well-defined radiolucency with bony septa, which divide the lesion into compartments of varying size. It can also have a honeycombed or soap bubble appearance. When small, it may be unilocular, round in shape and resemble an odontogenic cyst. An important radiological feature is resorption of the roots of the adjacent teeth.

The unicystic ameloblastoma typically occurs appears as a unilocular or locu-

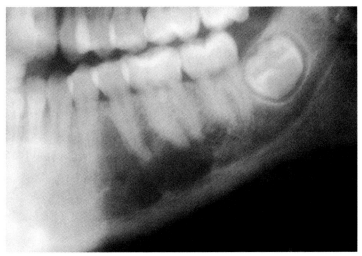

Fig 7-17 Solitary bone cyst extending from the lower first premolar to the lower second molar. Note how its upper margin arches upwards between the roots of the posterior teeth.

lated radiolucency often associated with the crown of an unerupted tooth and so resembles a dentigerous cyst. Some lesions reach a considerable size with marked expansion and thinning of the mandible, as shown in Fig 7-16.

Solitary (Traumatic) Bone Cyst
The aetiology of this condition is unknown, although at one time it was thought that it resulted from failure of organisation of a traumatically induced intramedullary haematoma. It has no epithelial lining and the term cyst refers to its radiographic appearance. Surgical exploration reveals an empty bony cavity. Once bleeding has been induced into the cavity by this procedure, the condition resolves.

Clinical features
Solitary bone cysts typically occur during the second decade of life, in the body of the mandible. It is usually asymptomatic and so is usually found as a chance radiographic finding.

Radiographic features
The solitary bone cyst appears as an ovoid, fairly well defined radiolucency in the body of the mandible. Typically, its superior margin is scalloped where it extends up between the roots of the teeth (Fig 7-17). Expansion of the

123

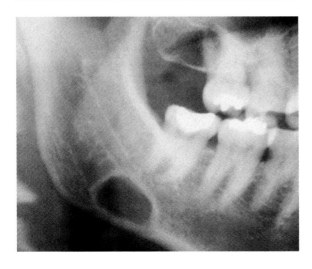

Fig 7-18 Stafne bone cavity.

bony cortex is unusual and, if present, is best demonstrated on an occlusal radiograph.

Stafne Bone Cavity
This is a depression on the lingual aspect of the mandible, the aetiology of which is poorly understood. It is uncommon and mainly affects men over 35 years of age. Being asymptomatic, it is discovered as an unexpected radiographic finding.

Radiographic features
The cavity is densely radiolucent, due to the loss of the lingual cortical plate. It is located below the inferior alveolar canal just anterior to the angle of the mandible, but sometimes occurs as far forwards as the lower second molar. It is oval in shape, rarely exceeds 2.0 cm, is well defined and, has a punched out appearance and often has a cortical margin, as shown in Fig 7-18.

Ill-Defined Radiolucencies of the Jaws

A radiolucency with an ill-defined margin indicates that the lesion is undergoing rapid change. It thus occurs with acute infections, such as osteomyelitis, and infiltrative malignant tumours.

Osteomyelitis
Osteomyelitis is inflammation of the marrow spaces. It arises as a complica-

tion of an odontogenic infection, e.g. apical abscess, or following the extraction of an infected tooth.

Clinical features
Osteomyelitis mainly affects the mandible. There is severe pain, often described as throbbing in nature. The infection invariably spreads to produce inflammatory swelling of the oral soft tissues and skin. Involvement of the inferior alveolar canal can result in numbness of the lower lip.

Radiological features
It takes about two weeks after the onset of inflammation before there is sufficient decalcification of the bone to be evident on a radiograph. Initially the bony trabeculae become thinned and appear indistinct so the affected bone becomes patchily radiolucent with ill-defined margins (Fig 7-19). The process leads to areas of bone necrosis (sequestra), which appear as irregularly shaped areas of bone surrounded by an ill-defined zone of radiolucency.

Malignant Tumours
Malignant tumours that affect the jaws may arise from:
- Local spread from tumours of the oral cavity, e.g. squamous cell carcinoma of the mouth and maxillary sinus. The former results in a saucerised bony cavity with moderate to ill-defined margins. Details of the latter are described on page 141.

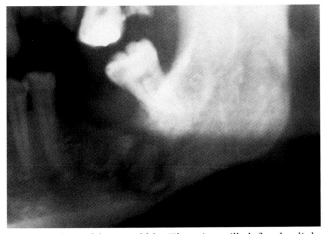

Fig 7-19 Osteomyelitis of the mandible. There is an ill-defined radiolucent in the body of the mandible in the premolar/molar region. It extends to the lower border of the mandible which has become thinned. Note the presence of sequestra, seen as radiopacities, within the radiolucency.

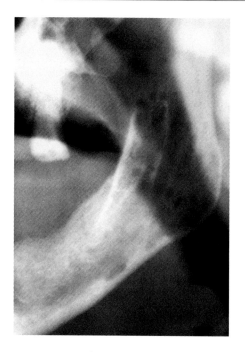

Fig 7-20 Metastatic deposits from breast carcinoma which appear as ill defined, irregularly radiolucencies in the left mandibular ramus and posterior lower cortex.

- Metastatic deposits tend to seed in areas of red bone marrow, thus jaw lesions occur the posterior body of the mandible. Many are painful and involvement of the inferior alveolar canal results in sensory loss to the lower lip. They produce bone destruction rather than bone resorption, so their radiographic appearance can resemble osteomyelitis. Most are lytic with ill-defined margins. However, some, e.g. from the prostate, may produce bone. The commonest primary sites are bronchus and breast (Fig 7-20).
- Primary tumours of bone, e.g. osteogenic sarcoma. These are rare but important lesions. Osteogenic sarcoma of the jaws produces variable amounts of bone and so may appear radiolucent and/or radiopaque. An important early feature is localised, irregular widening of the periodontal ligament space in the area of the tumour.

Mixed Density and Radiopaque Lesions of the Jaws

Jaw lesions appear radiopaque because of:
- excess formation of dental tissue
- excess formation of bone tissue
- dystrophic mineralisation
- metallic or other dense foreign material.

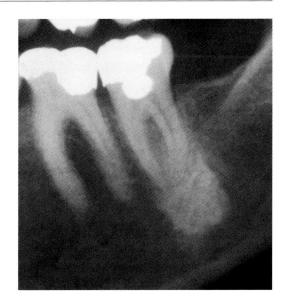

Fig 7-21 Sclerosing osteitis due to low-grade irritation from the roots of the lower left second molar.

Sclerosing Osteitis

This is a common condition that arises from low-grade chronic stimulation of the bone, from a non-vital or chronically inflamed tooth resulting in excess bone deposition. It is usually asymptomatic and so found as an incidental radiographic finding.

Radiographic features
Sclerosing osteitis appears as a periapical radiopacity heavily restored, carious or root-filled lower posterior tooth (Fig 7-21). The margins are irregular and abut against normal bone. There is no peripheral radiolucent capsular space, a feature that helps differentiate it from periapical cemento-osseous dysplasia.

Osteosclerosis (Dense Bone Island)

This condition has a similar appearance to that of sclerosing osteitis, except that the adjacent tooth or teeth are sound. It is mainly found in the premolar/molar region of the mandible as an irregularly shaped radiopacity of fairly uniform density (Fig 7-22).

Osteoma

There is some uncertainty whether osteomas are benign tumours of bone or hamartomas, as some show little or no growth. Osteomas are derived

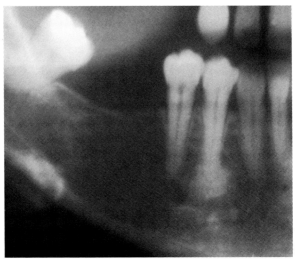

Fig 7-22 Osteosclerosis at the apex of the lower right second premolar.

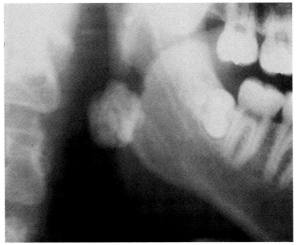

Fig 7-23 Compact osteoma at the angle of the mandible.

either from cancellous or compact bone, which is reflected in their radiographic appearance (Fig 7-23). They may be single entities, but multiple osteomas are a feature of familial adenomatous polyposis coli (Gardner's syndrome). This is an inherited condition in which there are multiple unerupted supernumerary and permanent teeth, skin lesions and prema-lignant polyps of the colon and congenital hypertrophy of retinal pigment epithelium (CHRPE).

Bony Tori and Bony Overgrowths
Bony tori and exostoses are developmental, localised areas of hyperplastic bone with limited growth potential. Mandibular tori may be single (torus), or multiple, unilateral, or more commonly bilateral, and are found on the lingual alveolus in the premolar region. The maxillary torus is more common, having an incidence of about 20%, and is located in the midline of the posterior half of the hard palate. Small tori are unlikely to show on a DPR. However, a large mandibular torus produces a fusiform radiopacity close to the alveolar crest in the premolar region.

Odontomes
An odontome is a hamartoma consisting of the dental tissues. There are two varieties:
• compound odontome
• complex odontome

Both types are often chance radiographic findings but may become noticed as they often impede the eruption of a tooth.

Radiographic features
Odontomes are dense structures due to the presence of enamel, dentine and cementum. The compound odontome most often develops in the upper ante-rior region of the jaws during childhood and consists of a collection of several small teeth (denticles) surrounded by a radiolucent capsule (Fig 7-24).

The complex odontome mainly occurs in the posterior region of the man-dible and contains dental tissues arranged haphazardly. When mature, it appears as a dense, mottled radiopacity that is well defined and surrounded by a thin radiolucent capsular space (Fig 7-25).

Fibrous Dysplasia
This condition occurs during childhood and presents as a painless bony expansion. The condition may affect one bone (monostotic) or more than one bone (polyostotic). It has a variable radiographic appearance which rarely may be radiolucent but typically is seen as a stippled, orange peel or ground glass radiopacity, the margins of which are poorly delineated.

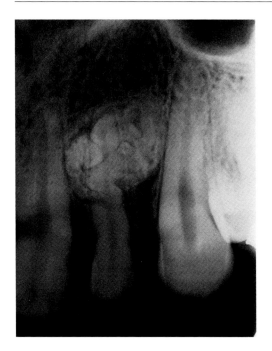

Fig 7-24 Compound odontome showing numerous denticles enclosed by a radiolucent capsular space.

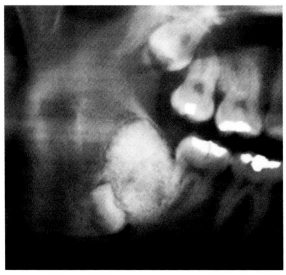

Fig 7-25 Part of a dental panoramic radiograph showing a complex odontome distal to the lower second molar. The wisdom tooth has been displaced inferiorly. Note the marked density of the odontome and the peripheral radiolucent capsular margin.

Cemento-Ossifying Lesions

This is a group of conditions in which bone is replaced by fibrous tissue, which then undergoes mineralisation. The histological differentiation between bone and cementum is difficult, so osseous and cementum-containing conditions are often considered together. The radiographic appearance depends on the relative amounts of fibrous and calcified tissue. The group consists of:

- periapical cemento-osseous dysplasia (PCD)
- florid cemento-osseous dysplasia (FCD)
- cemento-ossifying fibroma
- benign cementoblastoma (rare).

The first two are similar and are considered together.

Periapical Cemento-Osseous Dysplasia and Florid Cemento-Osseous Dysplasia

Clinical features

Both conditions are mainly found in women of Afro-Caribbean origin. They are asymptomatic and the involved teeth remain vital. The term 'florid' is used when the lesions are large and extensive.

Radiological features

The radiographic appearance depends on the relative proportions of fibrous and calcified tissue. The condition more commonly occurs in the mandible and is usually multiple, whilst solitary lesions are uncommon. Each lesion goes through three stages. Initially it is radiolucent and may resemble a periapical granuloma or radicular cyst (Fig 7-26a). However, more frequently the condition is not discovered until calcified tissue has been deposited usually centrally within the radiolucency to produce a mixed density appearance (Figs 7-26b and 7-27). In the final stage, the lesion becomes almost totally radiopaque, except for a thin radiolucent peripheral capsular space (Fig 7-26c).

Cemento-Ossifying Fibroma

Clinical features

This condition is regarded as an odontogenic neoplasm. It presents usually in young adults, mainly in the premolar and molar regions of the mandible. Females are affected more frequently than males. It tends to be slow growing, is usually asymptomatic, but can enlarge sufficiently to produce jaw expansion and become painful and tender.

131

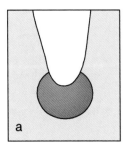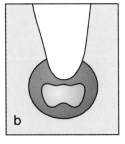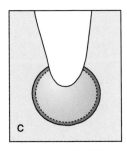

Fig 7-26 The three stages of periapical cemento-osseous dysplasia (PCD). a) The initial stage (stage I) of periapical cemento-osseous dysplasia (PCD). b) Stage II or the intermediate stage of PCD showing a mixed density appearance. c) Mature or stage III PCD with thin radiolucent peripheral capsular space.

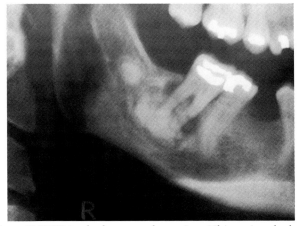

Fig 7-27 Stage II PCD in the lower molar region. This patient had several similar deposits throughout the mandibular alveolus.

Radiological features
This depends on the relative amounts of fibrous and calcified tissue. It may be largely radiolucent, but a careful examination may show wisps or coarse areas of calcification (Fig 7-28). Alternatively it may appear mainly radiopaque due to moderate to extensive amounts of calcification. Large lesions expand the bone, resulting in thinning and perforation of the bony cortex. The margin is well defined, which helps differentiate it from fibrous dysplasia.

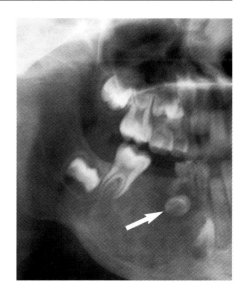

Fig 7-28 Cemento-ossifying fibroma of the mandible. There is a mixed density lesion extending from the incisor-canine region of the mandible to the molar region. There has been expansion of the lower border of the mandible and displacement of the developing permanent canine and premolar (arrowed) teeth.

Trauma

The DPR is widely used in the assessment of fractures of the mandible and condylar neck. However, in most cases a postero-anterior view is necessary, particularly if the fractures are displaced. Fractures of the mandible tend to occurs at specific sites, such as the angle or body, and contralateral fractures are common. A fracture in the parasymphyseal region is not always well shown on a DPR when an intra-oral radiograph may be indicated (Fig 7-29).

Trauma of the teeth is best assessed on intra-oral radiographs because of their better definition.

Disorders in the Soft Tissues

Salivary Duct Calculi
Salivary calculi are calcified deposits that form within the duct lumen, with most (80-90%) developing in the submandibular gland duct system and 10–20% associated with the parotid gland. Calculi may be single or multiple, and often develop at certain sites within the duct, e.g. at the duct orifice. They vary widely in size, from a millimetre to over a centimetre. Some are poorly mineralised and may not show on plain radiographs.

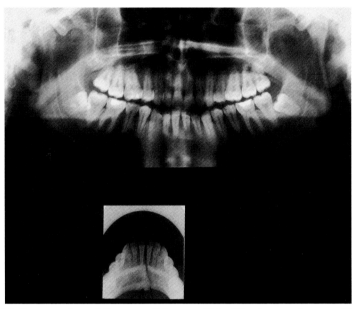

Fig 7-29 Parasymphyseal fracture of the mandible. The fracture is not evident on the DPR, but is clearly depicted in the occlusal views.

Clinical features
These may be:
- obstructive: recurrent swelling of the affected gland occurring at meal times, lasting minutes to hours
- persistent, painful swelling due to acute infection of the salivary gland (acute sialadenitis), particularly associated with reduced salivary flow
- no symptoms
- the patient may be able to feel the stone.

Radiographic features
The DPR is useful for showing calculi within the submandibular gland, but is not particularly helpful for detecting stones in the main part of the sub-mandibular or parotid duct because of superimposition of bone or teeth. Stones in the submandibular duct are better shown on a lower true occlu-sal. A large stone occupying much of the submandibular gland is shown in Fig 7-30.

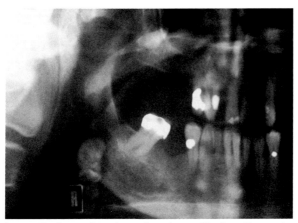

Fig 7-30 A large calculus within the right submandibular salivary gland.

Calcified Lymph Node

Calcified lymph nodes are usually asymptomatic and so detected unexpectedly on radiographs. Submandibular and cervical nodes can undergo dystrophic mineralisation following chronic infection with, for example, the TB bacterium. Typically, the calcified node has a radiopaque 'cauliflower' appearance due to the presence of numerous focal calcifications (Fig 7-31).

Tonsilloliths

Tonsilloliths are deposits of calcium salts within the palatine tonsillar crypts. They vary in size but generally appear as small radiopaque foci superimposed over the ramus of the mandible (Fig 7-32). They may be mistaken for parotid duct stones, but the location is different from tonsilloliths.

Foreign Bodies

Most foreign bodies are asymptomatic and, as a consequence, tend to be found as an incidental radiographic finding. Common examples include amalgam and extruded root filling material. A more unusual example is shown in Fig 7-33.

Disorders of the Maxillary Sinus

Disorders of the maxillary sinus may develop as a complication of dental disease or treatment, or due to primary disease of the paranasal sinuses.

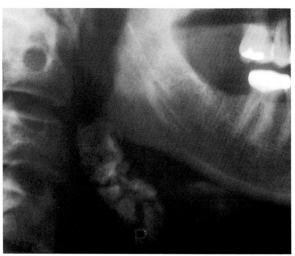

Fig 7-31 Marked dystrophic mineralisation of the cervical lymph nodes following infection with TB. Note its different position and orientation compared with the salivary calculus in Fig 7-29.

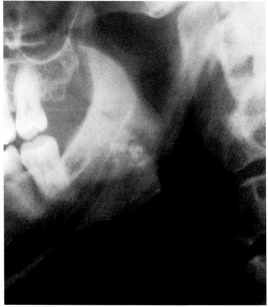

Fig 7-32 Tonsilloliths. Focal radiopaque collections within the tonsillar crypts.

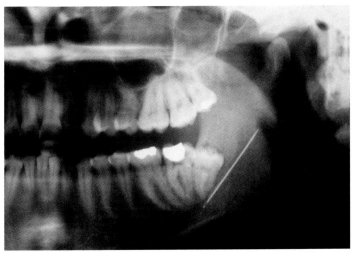

Fig 7-33 Sewing needle lying on the medial aspect of the mandible. The eye of the needle is visible just below the apex of the lower third molar.

Root Displaced Into the Maxillary Sinus

Clinical features

Root displacement is an uncommon complication of tooth extraction, but one that requires appropriate management. It is important to determine the location of the root. Initially this consists of a thorough clinical examination of the tooth socket and mouth. If a communication with the sinus is discovered, it is probable that it has been caused by the extraction procedure and that the root has been displaced into the sinus cavity, or more rarely that it lies just under the sinus lining.

Radiographic features

The radiographs that may display a root in the sinus are:
- periapical radiograph of the tooth socket
- upper oblique occlusal radiograph, centred over the tooth socket. This view shows more of the sinus than a periapical view but, given its angulation, is more distorted
- DPR.

A DPR is required to show a displaced root when it is not visible on an intraoral film (Fig 7-34). The root appears as a radiopacity against the radiolucent antral cavity. Identification of roots that lie distant from the socket can, how-

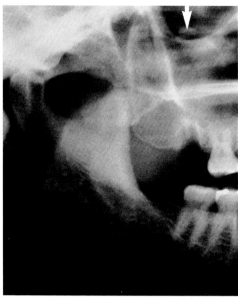

Fig 7-34 Root displaced in to the antrum and lying close to the antral roof (arrow).

ever, be difficult particularly if small and obscured by unwanted shadows such as the root of the zygoma when other imaging should be considered.

Oro-Antral Fistula (OAF)
This is an epithelial lined tract between the antral cavity and the mouth. It usually develops as a complication tooth extraction. However, a destructive condition of the maxilla or maxillary antrum should be considered in the absence of a recent extraction.

Clinical features
The size of the communication influences the clinical features. A narrow fistula may result in no symptoms, but if the sinus becomes infected because of, for example, the presence of a root in the antrum or because of poor drainage through the socket, the patient will develop features of a unilateral sinusitis. Alternatively a large communication may allow fluid from the mouth to enter the antrum and exit via the nose. Examination of the mouth shows lack of mucosal epithelialisation across the socket, which contains granulation tissue.

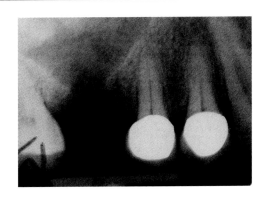

Fig 7-35 Oro-antral fistula following extraction of the upper first molar. Note the discontinuity of the antral floor

Radiographic features
Look for discontinuity of the bony outline of the floor of the antrum, as shown in Fig 7-35, and the presence of opacification of the antral cavity due to inflammatory swelling of the antral lining.

Root-Filling Material
Root-filling cement or sealant may inadvertently be displaced into the sinus cavity. Generally, this mishap does not result in discomfort, but should not be ignored. Consideration should be given to referral for a second opinion on its management.

Radiological features
Root-filling materials are radiopaque and appear as globules or focal radiopaque collections lying at varying distances from the site of displacement (Fig 7-36).

Mucous Cysts of the Maxillary Antrum
This condition is a relatively common. There are two types: inflammatory and retention cysts. It is thought that the former arises from cystic degeneration of chronically inflamed antral mucosa or an antral polyp, in which tissue fluid collects in clefts formed within the thickened antral lining. Retention cysts arise from obstruction of the ducts of the mucous glands found in the antral lining, leading to accumulation of fluid within the dilated ducts.

Clinical features
Mucous retention cysts are usually asymptomatic.

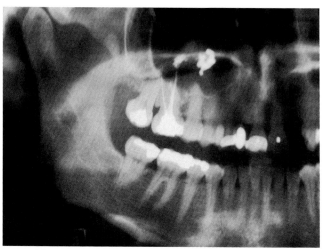

Fig 7-36 Root-filling cement lying within the antral cavity. There are several dense focal collections visible.

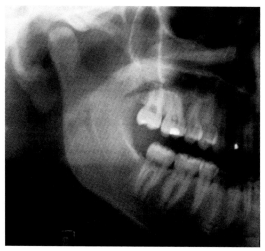

Fig 7-37 Antral mucous cyst producing a smooth domed shaped radiopacity above the posterior teeth. The bony floor of the sinus remains intact.

Radiographic features
A mucous retention cyst appears as smooth, dome-shaped radiopacity, of variable size, found most often on the floor of the maxillary antrum. The bony outline of the maxillary antrum remains intact and undisplaced, so it

is important that this outline can be traced. Because the mucous cyst arises from the antral lining and expands into the antral cavity, there is no bone on its upper margin as shown in Fig 7-37. However, odontogenic cysts that expand into the antrum can produce a similar dome-shaped opacity but display a thin layer of bone superiorly due to elevation of the antral floor as they expand from the alveolus.

Most mucous retention cysts resolve spontaneously. However, polyps, which can look similar, are often more persistent.

Carcinoma of the Maxillary Sinus
Clinical features
This tumour is uncommon. It mainly affects middle-aged or elderly men, and there appears to be an association with cigarette smoking and industrial airborne pollutants. Initially there are few symptoms whilst the tumour enlarges within the antral cavity. However, the dentist may be the first to see this condition, as early symptoms include intraoral swelling, tooth mobility, recurrent sinusitis and facial pain. Later features are due to nasal obstruction, involvement of the orbit or spread into infratemporal fossa. The condition has usually reached a considerable size by the time of detection.

Radiographic features
On a DPR there is destruction of the bony walls of the antrum, in particular the floor and posterior walls, the outlines of which become discontinuous (Fig 7-38). The affected antrum appears radiopaque due to the presence of the tumour mass. Involvement of the alveolar bone results in bone destruction around the teeth, which extends to the alveolar crest where a soft-tissue swelling may be evident.

Disorders of the Temporomandibular Joint

The commonest disorders that affect the TMJ are myofascial pain dysfunction syndrome (MPDS) and internal derangement; sometimes these conditions are considered under the heading of temporomandibular dysfunction (TMD). In MPDS there is tenderness of the muscles of mastication, whereas internal derangement is due to an abnormal disc position, usually associated with locking and clicking.

In TMD, the mandibular condyles do not show abnormal changes other than occasional functional remodelling, thus radiography is not routinely

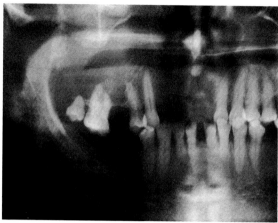

Fig 7-38 Carcinoma of the right maxillary antrum. There is erosion of the bony outline of the floor, tuberosity and posterior wall of the antral cavity (compare with the opposite side). The right antral cavity appears radiopaque due to the presence of the tumour.

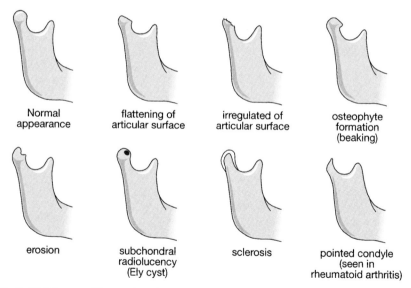

Normal appearance

flattening of articular surface

irregulated of articular surface

osteophyte formation (beaking)

erosion

subchondral radiolucency (Ely cyst)

sclerosis

pointed condyle (seen in rheumatoid arthritis)

Fig 7-39 Diagram illustrating the spectrum of appearances of condylar morphology following degenerative joint disease (osteoarthrosis). These include flattening, subchondral sclerosis, erosion and irregularity of the articular surface. An Ely cyst represents an area of degeneration. By contrast rheumatoid arthritis presents as an erosion of the posterior and anterior aspects of the condyle.

142

indicated in the vast majority of cases, unless the condition fails to respond to conventional therapy or the diagnosis is in doubt.

However, degenerative joint disease can produce symptoms similar to TMD, with the addition of grating, crepitus and tenderness of the temporomandibular joint. This condition produces a range of radiographic changes to the condylar head, including sclerosis, irregularity, erosion and flattening. While it could thus be argued that crepitus might be an indicator for radiography, this should only be the case where confirmation of this finding would be likely to influence patient management (Fig 7–39).

Further Reading

Brocklebank L. Dental Radiology. Oxford: Oxford University Press, 1997.

Chapple ILC and Gilbert AD. Quintessentials of Dental Practice 1-Understanding Periodontal Diseases: Assessment and Diagnostic Procedures in Practice. London: Quintessence, 2002.

Cawson RA and Odell EW. Oral Pathology and Oral Medicine. 7th Edn. Edinburgh: Churchill Livingstone, 1998.

Horner K, Rout J and Rushton VE. Quintessentials of Dental Practice 5- Interpreting Dental Radiographs. London: Quintessence, 2002.

Whaites E. Essentials of Dental Radiography and Radiology. 3rd Edn. Edinburgh: Churchill Livingstone, 2002.

White SC and Pharoah MJ. Oral Radiology 5th Edn. St. Louis: Mosby 2004.

Index

Quintessentials for General Dental Practitioners Series
in 50 volumes

Editor-in-Chief: Professor Nairn H F Wilson

General Dentistry, Editor: Nairn Wilson

Implantology in General Dental Practice	available
Culturally Sensitive Oral Healthcare	available
Dental Erosion	available
Managing Orofacial Pain in Practice	Autumn 2006
Dental Bleaching	Autumn 2006
Special Care Dentistry	Autumn 2006
Infection Control for the Dental Team	Spring 2007
Therapeutics and Medical Emergencies in the Everyday Clinical Practice of Dentistry	Spring 2007

Oral Surgery and Oral Medicine, Editor: John G Meechan

Practical Dental Local Anaesthesia	available
Practical Oral Medicine	available
Practical Conscious Sedation	available
Minor Oral Surgery in Dental Practice	available

Imaging, Editor: Keith Horner

Interpreting Dental Radiographs	available
Panoramic Radiology	available
Twenty-first Century Dental Imaging	Autumn 2006

Periodontology, Editor: Iain L C Chapple

Understanding Periodontal Diseases: Assessment and Diagnostic Procedures in Practice	available
Decision-Making for the Periodontal Team	available
Successful Periodontal Therapy – A Non-Surgical Approach	available
Periodontal Management of Children, Adolescents and Young Adults	available
Periodontal Medicine: A Window on the Body	available

Endodontics, Editor: John M Whitworth

Rational Root Canal Treatment in Practice	available
Managing Endodontic Failure in Practice	available
Restoring Endodontically Treated Teeth	Autumn 2006

Prosthodontics, Editor: P Finbarr Allen

Teeth for Life for Older Adults	available
Complete Dentures – from Planning to Problem Solving	available
Removable Partial Dentures	available
Fixed Prosthodontics in Dental Practice	available
Occlusion: A Theoretical and Team Approach	Autumn 2006

Operative Dentistry, Editor: Paul A Brunton

Decision-Making in Operative Dentistry	available
Aesthetic Dentistry	available
Communicating in Dental Practice	available
Indirect Restorations	Summer 2006
Choosing and Using Dental Materials	Autumn 2006

Paediatric Dentistry/Orthodontics, Editor: Marie Therese Hosey

Child Taming: How to Cope with Children in Dental Practice	available
Paediatric Cariology	available
Treatment Planning for the Developing Dentition	available
Managing Dental Trauma in Practice	available

General Dentistry and Practice Management, Editor: Raj Rattan

The Business of Dentistry	available
Risk Management	available
Quality Matters: From Clinical Care to Customer Service	Summer 2006
Practice Management for the Dental Team	Autumn 2006
Dental Practice Design	Autumn 2006
Handling Complaint in Dental Practice	Autumn 2006

Dental Team, Editor: Mabel Slater

Team Players in Dentistry	Autumn 2006

Quintessence Publishing Co. Ltd., London